Qualitative Research in Evidence-Based Rehabilitation

Commissioning editor: Susan Young
Project development manager: Jane Dingwall/Pat Miller
Project manager: Jane Dingwall
Design direction: Judith Wright
Illustration manager: Bruce Hogarth

Qualitative Research in Evidence-Based Rehabilitation

Edited by

Karen Whalley Hammell PhD MSc OT(C) DipCOT
Researcher and Writer, Oxbow, Saskatchewan, Canada

Christine Carpenter PhD MA BA DipPT
Senior Instructor, Division of Physical Therapy, School of Rehabilitation Sciences, University of British Columbia, Vancouver, Canada

Foreword by

Susan R Harris PhD PT
Professor, School of Rehabilitation Sciences, Faculty of Medicine, University of British Columbia, Vancouver, Canada

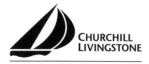

EDINBURGH LONDON NEW YORK OXFORD PHILADELPHIA ST LOUIS SYDNEY TORONTO 2004

CHURCHILL LIVINGSTONE
An imprint of Elsevier Limited

First published 2004

ISBN 0 443 07231 0

British Library Cataloguing in Publication Data
A catalogue record for this book is available from the British Library

Library of Congress Cataloging in Publication Data
A catalog record for this book is available from the Library of Congress

Printed in China

Contents

Contributors

Christine Carpenter PhD MA BA DipPT
*Senior Instructor, Division of Physical Therapy,
School of Rehabilitation Sciences, University of
British Columbia, Vancouver, Canada*

Chris was educated as a physiotherapist in
Liverpool, England, and attained her graduate
degrees at the University of British Columbia,
Canada, in Educational Studies. Dr Carpenter
has received several university teacher of
excellence awards. Her teaching interests
include interdisciplinary healthcare ethics,
communication, physical therapy procedures,
qualitative research methodology, and
rehabilitation theory and practice. An editor/
author of *Using Qualitative Research: A Practical
Introduction for Occupational and Physical Therapists*
(2000), her current research initiatives are focused
on the long-term experience of spinal cord
injury.

Deborah J. Corring DipOT MSc OTReg(Ont)
*Doctoral candidate and Programme Co-Leader,
Regional Mental Health Care St Thomas, St Joseph's
Health Care, London, Ontario, Canada*

Deb received her Diploma in Occupational
Therapy from Queen's University, Ontario, and
worked as a clinician and administrator in the
mental health service sector. Her MSc research
documented a client definition of client-centred
care. After graduation she continued to explore
client perspectives on issues such as quality of
life, leisure, work, independent living and
satisfaction with services. She is currently
pursuing a doctorate in rehabilitation sciences,
focusing on client perspectives pertaining to
definitions of quality of life.

Michael Curtin MPhil BOccThy SROT
*Lecturer in Occupational Therapy, School of Health
Professions and Rehabilitation Sciences, University
of Southampton, UK*

Since graduating from the University of
Queensland, Michael has worked as an
occupational therapist in Australia, Botswana
and England, predominantly in the fields of
paediatrics and spinal cord lesions. He currently
enjoys lecturing and working with
undergraduate students. Of his various
publications, Michael is proudest of the two
co-written books, one on cerebral palsy and the
other on spinal cord injury, collaboratively
funded by the World Health Organization,
World Federation of Occupational Therapy and
World Confederation for Physical Therapy. The
Department of Health funded the investigation
described in this book. His current passion is the
use of auto/biographical research techniques
with disabled children.

Jan Gwyer PhD PT
*Associate Clinical Professor, Division of Physical
Therapy, Duke University School of Medicine,
Durham, North Carolina, USA*

Dr Gwyer holds a bachelor of science degree
from the Medical College of Virginia and
master's and doctor of philosophy degrees from

the University of North Carolina at Chapel Hill. Jan has held several leadership roles in the American Physical Therapy Association and serves as a consultant in the areas of clinical education and career paths in physical therapy. She teaches doctor of physical therapy students and clinicians in the area of evidence-based practice.

Laurita M. Hack PhD MBA PT FAPTA
Professor and Chair, Department of Physical Therapy, Temple University, Philadelphia, Pennsylvania, USA

Dr Hack received her BSc degree from Wilmington College and her MS degree (in physical therapy) from Case Western Reserve University, USA. She also received an MBA in health care from the Wharton School and a PhD from the School of Education, both at the University of Pennsylvania. She has provided clinical care through her own practice. Laurita has thoroughly enjoyed the personal and professional growth that working with her colleagues on the project described in this book has allowed.

Karen Whalley Hammell PhD MSc OT(C) DipCOT
Researcher and Writer, Oxbow, Saskatchewan, Canada

Karen is an occupational therapist who earned her MSc (with Distinction) from the University of Southampton, UK, and her PhD in interdisciplinary studies (rehabilitation sciences, anthropology, sociology) from the University of British Columbia, Canada. Dr Hammell is the author of *Spinal Cord Injury Rehabilitation* (1995), an editor/author of *Using Qualitative Research: A Practical Introduction for Occupational and Physical Therapists* (2000), the author of several book chapters and a member of the editorial board of *Spinal Cord*. Her research interests include spinal cord injury, quality of life issues, disability theory (equality of life issues) and the dynamics of client–professional power (e.g. client-centred practice and research).

Emily Jaramazovic BSc MSc CAES
Freelance Research Consultant, Southampton, UK

Since gaining her degrees in sociology, Emily has been involved in a wide variety of qualitative research projects. Her main research interest is in the sexual health of young people and international seafarers. For the duration of the evidence-based practice research described in this book, Emily was employed part-time at the School of Health Professions and Rehabilitation Sciences, University of Southampton. As well as freelance research work, she is currently employed part-time as an Outreach Worker providing information and support to women in the commercial sex industry.

Gail M. Jensen PhD PT FAPTA
Associate Dean for Faculty Development and Assessment; Professor of Physical Therapy, School of Pharmacy and Health Professions; and Faculty Associate, Center for Health Policy and Ethics, Creighton University, Omaha, Nebraska, USA

Dr Jensen holds a BSc degree in education from the University of Minnesota, an MA in physical therapy and a PhD in educational evaluation/sociology – both from Stanford University. Her research interests, publications and presentations span the areas of clinical reasoning, development of expertise, qualitative research, and interprofessional education and assessment. She has collaborated on six books, has served on several editorial boards, and is currently deputy editor of *Physiotherapy Research International*.

Mary Law PhD OT(C)

Professor, Associate Dean (Health Sciences) and Director of the School of Rehabilitation Science, McMaster University, and Co-Director of CanChild Centre for Childhood Disability Research, Hamilton, Ontario, Canada

Dr Law is an occupational therapist with graduate training in epidemiology, and health and social planning. Her research interests include the development, validation and transfer into practice of outcome measures; evaluation of family-centred interventions for children with disabilities; and the study of environmental, family and child factors that affect the participation of children with disabilities. Mary has written books on client-centred occupational therapy and evidence-based rehabilitation.

Karen Rebeiro BScOT MScOT
Clinical Researcher, Northeast Mental Health Centre, Sudbury, Ontario, Canada

Karen obtained her BSc in occupational therapy in 1985 and her MSc in occupational therapy in 1997, both from the University of Western Ontario, Canada. She has worked in the field of mental health for the past 17 years. For the last 6 years she has worked as a clinical researcher for the Northeast Mental Health Centre in collaboration with mental health consumers, endeavouring to understand their experiences and thereafter to influence policy and systemic issues that prohibit consumers' active participation in the community.

Candice Schachter DipPT BA MHK PhD
Associate Professor, School of Physical Therapy, University of Saskatchewan, Saskatoon, Canada

Dr Schachter trained as a physical therapist at the University of Saskatchewan and completed her graduate education at the University of Windsor and the University of Western Ontario. Her main areas of interest are physical activity for clinical populations and client-centred practice. Candice continues to work with colleagues examining client-centred care for adults who have experienced violence in their lives and is also conducting research in the area of fibromyalgia and exercise.

Katherine Shepard PhD PT FAPTA
Professor and Director of the PhD programme in Physical Therapy, Temple University, Philadelphia, Pennsylvania, USA

Katherine Shepard received a BSc degree in psychology (1962) from Hood College, a BS degree in physical therapy (1963) from Ithaca

College, MS degrees in both physical therapy (1969) and sociology (1976), and a PhD in sociology of education (1978) from Stanford University. Dr Shepard has published over 60 articles and book chapters predominantly in the areas of social science research related to physical therapy practice and education. She is a co-author and co-editor (with Gail Jensen) of *Handbook of Teaching for Physical Therapists*, second edition (2002) and *Expertise in Physical Therapy Practice* (1999). She has received several awards for teaching excellence.

Carol Stalker RSW MSW PhD

Associate Professor, Faculty of Social Work, Wilfrid Laurier University, Waterloo, Ontario, Canada

Dr Stalker received her MSW from Wilfrid Laurier University, and her PhD in social work from Smith College, Northampton, Massachusetts. Carol has worked for over 20 years as a clinical social worker, primarily in mental health settings. Since 1985, she has worked extensively with women survivors of childhood sexual abuse, both individually and in group treatment. She has also conducted research evaluating clinical interventions with survivors, and investigating conditions that affect adult functioning in the aftermath of childhood trauma.

Melinda Suto BS(OT) MA(OT)
Doctoral Candidate and Senior Instructor, School of Rehabilitation Sciences, University of British Columbia, Vancouver, Canada

Melinda was educated in California, earning a bachelor's degree at San Jose State University and a master's degree at the University of Southern California. Before joining the School of Rehabilitation Sciences, she worked extensively with clients experiencing mental health problems. Melinda is completing her PhD in educational studies at the University of British Columbia. Her doctoral research focuses on leisure meanings created by women who immigrate to Canada and their participation in leisure activities. Other interests include a broad range of community mental health issues, conceptual development in occupational therapy, and informed shared decision-making.

Eli Teram PhD

Professor, Faculty of Social Work, Wilfrid Laurier University, Waterloo, Ontario, Canada

Eli has interdisciplinary education in social work and management. He received his education from Tel Aviv University, Israel, and McGill University, Montreal, Canada. His main areas of interest are the organizational interdisciplinary and interorganizational contexts of professionals' practice. For the past 25 years, Eli has been involved in teaching and conducting qualitative research employing a variety of research methods including interviews, participant observation, focus groups and participatory methods.

Foreword

Just as qualitative research studies are generally more interesting to read than most quantitative studies, so is this qualitative research text more readable and refreshing than many, standard quantitative methods texts. Drs Hammell and Carpenter, an occupational therapist and a physiotherapist by training, have done a superb job of integrating qualitative studies into an evidence-based framework that will be useful to rehabilitation researchers, practitioners, and students.

The editors have succeeded in inviting both an interdisciplinary and international group of authors, all of whom are established leaders in qualitative research relating to rehabilitation. The authors represent physiotherapists, occupational therapists, and social workers from Canada, Great Britain, and the United States, many of whom have integrated the results of their own studies within their respective chapters. The participants in those nine studies are equally diverse, representing expert physiotherapist clinicians, adults with mental illness, children with physical disabilities and adults with spinal cord injuries among others.

Sackett et al's most recent definition of evidence-based medicine requires the integration of *best research evidence* with *clinical expertise* and *patient values* (Sackett et al 2000). The inclusion of the patient's experience and values is an integral component of qualitative health research but is too often missing in quantitative studies. By including patients or clients of rehabilitation as participants or co-researchers, rather than as subjects to be studied by others, qualitative research directly encompasses patient values into the design and execution of those studies.

My own experience as a cancer patient highlights the importance of both quantitative and qualitative research in contributing to my own evidence-based decision-making. While the results of recent quantitative studies, including randomized controlled trials, greatly influenced my decisions in making informed choices about various chemotherapy combinations and appropriate sites for radiation, my own values as a patient (combined with evidence-based knowledge) mitigated my use and exploration of a whole host of alternative treatments to which many cancer patients routinely turn.

As a cancer patient, I became involved in both quantitative and qualitative studies, as a subject and as a participant, respectively. I believe that the results of *both* types of studies have contributed to my well being as a cancer survivor and have added to the evidence underlying and supporting cancer care for other patients and survivors.

Similarly, qualitative research provides essential 'evidence' in enhancing the well being and quality of life for individuals involved in rehabilitation. *Qualitative Research in Evidence-Based Rehabilitation* provides an important first step in informing rehabilitation practice through the results of qualitative studies. By integrating examples of the studies themselves within the chapters of this book, practitioners and students will be introduced to primary sources of evidence embedded within this seminal secondary source which, I suspect, will provide a very effective learning strategy.

Evidence has been defined as 'an outward sign' or 'something that furnishes proof' (Webster's Seventh New Collegiate Dictionary 1963). Qualitative research, as outlined by Carpenter in Chapter 1, commonly uses methods such as 'individual, in-depth interviewing, participant observation, and focus groups' and, by its very nature, is philosophically compatible with a client-centred ethic (see p. 10). It is abundantly clear that the patient's own voice, as captured in interviews or focus groups within qualitative research, provides an important 'outward sign' of that individual's response and adjustment to their own illness or disability.

The patient's or family's own interpretation of the impact of the disability on their lives is perhaps much more important 'proof' or evidence in informing practice than the biomedical aspects of the disability or impairment. Let me share an example from my own clinical experience as a paediatric physiotherapist to highlight that important difference. Two little girls with multiple and profound congenital disabilities come each year, with their parents, to 'guest lecture' in my paediatric neurorehabilitation course. Both have significant feeding difficulties. One of the girls has had a gastrostomy tube implanted to provide most of her nutritional needs since shortly after birth. It is her parents' fondest dream that she will learn to eat orally so that she will no longer have to be 'fed' through the tube. The other child, now 6 years old, recently had a gastrostomy tube put in place to enhance her nutrition. Her mother's response is that this tube is the 'greatest thing since sliced bread' because it makes feeding her

daughter easier and ensures that she is receiving adequate nutrition.

From an evidence-based, biomedical perspective, both little girls were candidates for supplemental nutrition and the gastrostomy tube was the appropriate scientific choice for each of them. Based on their families' values, however, the tube is a blessing for one child's family and a burden for the other's. By conducting in-depth interviewing of each of these families, a qualitative researcher would uncover the profound differences in their responses to this biomedical measure. This type of additional 'evidence' could then be used to enhance further decision-making about meeting the future nutritional needs of these two little girls, in concert with their families' values.

As the editors and chapter authors of *Qualitative Research in Evidence-Based Rehabilitation* have demonstrated so eloquently, there is clearly a need for *both* types of evidence in ensuring that the needs of rehabilitation clients and their families are being appropriately addressed. The rehabilitation world is considerably richer now as a result of publication of this important text. It is my fondest hope that this book will be embraced by rehabilitation practitioners and students as they strive to provide service that is both evidence-based *and* client-centred.

Vancouver 2003   Susan R Harris

REFERENCES

Sackett D, Strauss S, Richardson W, Rosenberg W, Haynes R 2000 Evidence-based medicine. How to practice and teach EBM. 2nd edn. Churchill Livingstone, Edinburgh
Random House Webster's Dictionary, 4th edn. 2001. Ballantine Books, New York

Preface

As a response to consumer demands for effective and relevant rehabilitation practice that is informed by research, government policies and professional guidelines are insisting that occupational therapy and physical therapy should be 'evidence based'. However, current variations in both interventions and models of service delivery suggest that considerable work needs to be done in occupational therapy and physical therapy to establish a coherent evidence base to support their practice. Further, it is evident that the theories that underpin these professions also suffer from a dearth of supportive research evidence.

Critics have suggested that traditional reliance upon quantitative methods of research by the rehabilitation professions has contributed to the apparent theory–practice gap, wherein the research that was undertaken had little or no relevance to the realities of clinical practice. In response, qualitative research methods are increasingly being adopted to generate relevant and useful knowledge with which to inform occupational and physical therapy practice.

Qualitative Research in Evidence-Based Rehabilitation draws upon qualitative research undertaken by an international group of researchers – working in Canada, Britain and the USA – who represent the professions of both occupational therapy and physical therapy. Through their research examples, the 15 authors illustrate how research questions arise from everyday practice and how qualitative methods permit findings to be grounded in the views of clients – thus assuring both relevance and usefulness. The authors demonstrate how the evidence generated from their studies was used: to critique and develop theory, to inform clinical practice, to influence the development of services that were responsive to clients' needs, and to provide a sound knowledge base for education, research and professional development. Research evidence provided not just knowledge, but change.

The aim of the book is to provide a thorough interrogation of the concept of evidence-based practice for the professions of occupational and physical therapy, demonstrating that this is a more complex requirement than a simple utilization of research. It achieves this by exploring simultaneously real research examples and those dimensions of professional practice that were informed by the research evidence.

The book will be useful for undergraduate and graduate students in physical and occupational therapy, educators, researchers, administrators and those clinicians who seek to ground their own practice in a sound evidence base.

This is a book that addresses one of the most prescient issues facing the rehabilitation professions today by providing elucidation not solely of the 'problem' of evidence-based practice but also of real responses.

Karen Whalley Hammell
Christine Carpenter

Oxbow, Saskatchewan and Vancouver,
December 2002

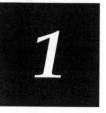

1

The contribution of qualitative research to evidence-based practice

Chris Carpenter

KEY POINTS

evidence-based practice; clinical expertise; theoretical knowledge; client knowledge; outcomes and effectiveness research; client-centred practice; qualitative methodologies and methods

OVERVIEW

This first chapter sets the stage for discussions in subsequent chapters of the various contributions that qualitative research can make to evidence-based practice in rehabilitation. Chris Carpenter traces the evolution of the evidence-based movement in medicine and defines its application to evidence-based practice in rehabilitation. Drawing on contemporary literature in medicine, occupational therapy and physiotherapy, she explores the limitations inherent in the concept of evidence-based practice and attributes these to the uncritical adoption of the quantitative research paradigm. Reflecting the concerns of physiotherapists working in rehabilitation settings who participated in her doctoral research, Chris discusses the lack of congruence between standardized outcome measures and effectiveness research in rehabilitation with the experience of clients with disability in their 'real' contexts, and with client-centred practice.

The dimensions of evidence-based practice – the 'best' available evidence, clinical expertise and client knowledge – are defined. Chris concludes the chapter by making the argument that qualitative research has an important role to fulfil in ensuring that all three dimensions are incorporated and equally valued in guiding theory building, directing and evaluating service and programme provision, and developing and implementing relevant and effective interventions.

INTRODUCTION

Evidence-based practice is 'a significant movement of fundamental importance in the delivery of health-care throughout the developing world' (Bithell 2000, p. 58). It represents an expansion of the concept of evidence-based medicine to encompass more aspects of health care, including rehabilitation (Law 2002). Evidence-based practice, according to the Council of Directors of Physical Therapy Academic Programs & the Canadian Physiotherapy Association (1995), has a theoretical body of knowledge, and uses the best available scientific evidence in clinical decision-making and standardized outcome measures to evaluate the care provided. The Canadian Association of Occupational Therapists et al (1999) define evidence-based occupational therapy as 'client-centered enablement of occupation based on client information and a critical review of relevant research, expert consensus and past experience' (p. 267). The rehabilitation disciplines have willingly subscribed to the evidence-based practice movement and its culture of accountability. As a consequence, evidence-based practice has emerged as one of the most influential concepts in the past decade, as apparent in the proliferation of textbooks and articles on the topic in both occupational therapy and physiotherapy (e.g. Bury & Mead 1998, Finch et al 2002, Law 2002, Taylor 2000). However, 'best' evidence is still primarily associated with 'scientific' evidence derived from experimental quantitative research, and rarely is appraisal of qualitative research findings considered a part of this process.

Increasingly, it is being recognized in medicine and the rehabilitation sciences that this pronounced emphasis on 'scientific' method reflects the assumptions, values and beliefs that characterize the dominant biomedical model (Miller & Crabtree 2000). Within this model, the need for rehabilitation services is indicated because the patient has some normative deviation in everyday functioning and it is assumed that the cause of the difficulty can be detected and measured objectively using standardized instruments and biomedical technology (Baum & Christiansen 1997). A number of healthcare disciplines, for example occupational therapy (Law 1998) and nursing (Carse & Nelson 1996), have developed theoretical interpretations of practice that go beyond the biomedical approach. This has been achieved by developing theories of professional practice that are interpreted and elaborated in practice and focused on the guiding principles of client-centred and holistic health care. Physiotherapy has been characterized by the profession's close alignment with medicine and its enthusiastic commitment to a positivist knowledge base. The central idea of positivism is that one can only be certain, or positive, of knowledge that is verifiable through measurement and observation. The reliance on observation is also defined as 'empiricism'. Positivism is based on the assumption that the mind and body are distinct, and makes the claim that an objective world (or reality) exists outside subjective human perceptions. It is the theoretical basis for the quantitative approach to research, which has become the 'received view' or the traditional method of science. At the beginning of this chapter I introduced the definitions of evidence-based practice developed by occupational therapy and physiotherapy. These clearly differentiate the philosophical orientations of the two professions, and illustrate physiotherapy's alignment with the 'scientific' approach. However, the absence of conceptual models or frameworks linking research to the *realities* of physiotherapy practice – the theory–practice gap – is beginning to be recognized within the profession (De Souza 1998, Roskell et al 1998).

Tensions are emerging between the imperative of evidence-based practice and the philosophies of practice of the rehabilitation disciplines (Hammell 2001). The focus on the 'scientific' method has resulted in clinicians being 'confronted by a growing body of information, much [of which] is invalid or irrelevant to clinical practice' (Rosenberg & Donald 1995, p. 1122). As a result, the need to broaden the definition of 'best' evidence and to address the 'missing evidences' needed to inform and support the complexities of practice (Miller & Crabtree 2000) is being increasingly articulated in the rehabilitation literature (Bithell 2000, Ritchie 2001, Sumsion 1997, Townsend & Rebeiro 2001). These calls for greater methodological diversity are beginning to be answered, and according to Miller & Crabtree (2000) 'the use of qualitative methods and multiple [research] paradigms is expanding, but such endeavours are still only patchwork, found more in the tributaries of clinical research than in the mainstream' (p. 609).

Sackett et al (2000), major proponents of evidence-based medicine, acknowledge that often the patient–clinician interaction is based on questions that relate to the patient's experience and understanding of disease or disability, diagnostic tests and treatments, rather than on the actual test results or measurable health outcomes. These authors acknowledge that 'qualitative research' provides an approach by which these issues can be explored. However, they clearly state that 'whilst we regard the integration of qualitative research to be one of the major current challenges in evidence-based medicine, we readily admit that we are not expert in this field and defer to others' (p. 21). *Qualitative Research in Evidence-Based Rehabilitation* represents our effort to recognize and explicate the important contribution that qualitative research can make in investigating the central and complex issues of rehabilitation practice and service delivery.

In this chapter I will review the emergence of evidence-based medicine and its meaning and implementation in rehabilitation. The limits and constraints of evidence-based practice as identified in the literature will be discussed in relation to the realities of rehabilitation practice and the degree of congruency with client-centred philosophies of practice. This chapter will provide an overview of how qualitative research 'evidence' can address contemporary concerns about accountability and the provision of best practice. In this way, it will frame the research examples and

discussions provided by the contributors of the ensuing chapters.

EVIDENCE-BASED MEDICINE

Evidence-based medicine (EBM) evolved from a problem-based learning strategy developed at McMaster University, Canada (Evidence-Based Working Group 1992), in which valid sources of knowledge were located and critically evaluated to aid rational decision-making. In 1996, Sackett et al defined evidence-based medicine as 'the conscientious, explicit, and judicious use of current best evidence in making decisions about the care of individual patients. The practice of evidence-based medicine means integrating individual clinical expertise with the best available external clinical evidence from systematic research' (p. 30). A more detailed definition provided by Rosenberg & Donald (1995) stated that EBM is 'the process of systematically finding, appraising, and using contemporaneous research findings as a basis for clinical decisions. Evidence-based medicine asks questions, finds and appraises the relevant data, and harnesses that information for everyday clinical practice' (p. 1122).

These definitions appeared to 'de-emphasize' alternative forms of medical knowledge, such as clinical expertise and experience or the patient's goals and opinions (Bury & Mead 1998), and have been challenged within medicine (Maynard 1997, Naylor 1995, Tanenbaum 1999, Tonelli 1998). In 2000, Sackett et al redefined evidence-based medicine as 'the integration of *best research evidence* with *clinical expertise* and *patient values*' (p. 1). This definition clearly acknowledges the important role of clinical experience, clinical wisdom and intuition in making use of the 'best' evidence in meeting 'the unique preferences, concerns and expectations each patient brings to the clinical encounter' (Sackett et al 2000, p. 1). In this latest iteration, 'best research evidence' has been expanded to emphasize the importance of 'patient-centred clinical research' (p. 1). However, the hierarchical evaluation of evidence continues to be based primarily on clearly defined levels of evidence resulting from optimally conducted experimental studies (Table 1.1). The randomized

Table 1.1 Levels of evidence (based on Sackett et al 2000, pp. 17–21)

Level	Type of evidence
I	Evidence from at least one systematic review (with homogeneity) of multiple randomized controlled trials
II	Evidence from systematic review of cohort studies (including at least one randomized controlled trial)
III	Evidence from systematic review (with homogeneity) of case–control studies or individual case–control studies
IV	Evidence from well designed case series (and poor-quality cohort and case–control studies)
V	Expert opinion without explicit critical appraisal or based on physiology, bench research or 'first principles'

Box 1.1 Objections to evidence-based practice

- It is too time consuming.
- There is not enough evidence.
- The evidence is not of sufficiently high quality.
- Clinicians lack the skills to differentiate between high- and low-quality studies.
- Clinical research does not provide certainty when it is most needed.
- Research findings cannot be applied to individual patients.
- Clinical research does not tell us about patients' individual experiences.
- It removes responsibility for decision-making from individual therapists.

controlled trial (RCT) continues to be viewed as the 'gold standard' among designs used to evaluate clinical interventions. As Tonelli (1998) suggests, evidence-based medicine is a logical development of the traditional medical model approach to patient care in which the emphasis is on isolating the cause and effecting a cure.

Primary criticisms of evidence-based medicine are based on the perception that clinical expertise is undervalued and that reliance on rigorous experimental research designs leads to neglect of the 'many smaller-ticket items in routine practice' (Naylor 1995, p. 840).

DEFINING EVIDENCE-BASED PRACTICE IN REHABILITATION

The same criticisms have been levelled at evidence-based practice in rehabilitation (Bithell 2000, Sumsion 1997). Herbert et al (2001) systematically enumerate these objections (Box 1.1) but join other rehabilitation authors (e.g. Law 2002, Taylor 2000) in refuting them. They argue that these objections are outweighed by the potential benefits of evidence-based practice, and that it is an approach to practice and teaching that facilitates research planning and the generation of new clinical knowledge.

Law (2002) addresses the myth that evidence-based practice is 'devoid of the need for individual clinical judgement' and that 'clinical expertise is irrelevant' (p. 6) by referring to the assertion of Sackett et al (1996) that 'external clinical evidence can inform, but never replace, individual clinical expertise. [This] expertise will assist the practitioner in deciding whether the external evidence applies to the individual client at all and, if so, how it should be integrated into a clinical decision' (p. 73). Law suggests that the effective integration of evidence-based practice is dependent on rehabilitation clinicians developing and combining the skills of awareness, consultation, judgement and creativity. In her view, the implementation of these four concepts will achieve the goal of 'focused awareness' or knowledge of how to access and judge the strength of evidence that bears on specific practice. In addition, by engaging in a consultative process, clinicians will be able to distil information from the findings of others and use the information to educate clients.

In my experience, the arguments posited by these authors in response to many of the concerns raised about evidence-based practice over the past decade are both compelling and generally accepted and understood by rehabilitation clinicians. Few occupational therapists or physiotherapists would argue with Banja's (1997) assertion that, without recourse to research evidence, clients are reliant upon the therapist's 'best guess' or 'whim' (p. 53), upon increasingly out-of-date primary education or a therapist's overinterpretation of the benefits of a therapeutic modality.

Over the past decade there has been a proliferation of occupational therapy and physiotherapy literature explaining and debating the concept of evidence-based practice. Both professions clearly subscribe to Law's (2002) claim that if 'evidence-based practice can be incorporated into the practitioner's repertoire, the professions will see a shift toward a more analytical, certain, and ultimately effective clinical practice in health care' (p. 8).

In a recent research study (Carpenter 2002), in which I explored dilemmas of practice in rehabilitation settings as experienced by physiotherapists, it was clear that the participants all perceived the need to justify their practice as part of their professional responsibility. They exhibited many of the skills essential to evidence-based practitioners. However, they articulated dilemmas associated with evidence-based practice that have not been addressed adequately by proponents of the concept. These dilemmas arose from the biomedical orientation of disability outcomes assessment and effectiveness research, and the perceived tension between the client-centred and evidence-based approaches to practice. These issues are the focus of a burgeoning debate in the healthcare literature about the limitations inherent in the narrow definition of evidence upon which clinical decisions are ostensibly based in evidence-based practice (Miller & Crabtree 2000, Ritchie 2001).

LIMITS OF EVIDENCE-BASED PRACTICE

Rehabilitation outcomes and effectiveness research

'Outcomes are the variables or issue of interest to the [clinician or] researcher. They represent factors that identify the results of interventions for example, functional health status, morbidity, mortality, quality of life, satisfaction, and cost' (Nicholson 2002, p. 214). Healthcare outcomes form the basis for decision-making and service provision, and are pivotal to evidence-based practice (Taylor 2000). The dilemma for the physiotherapists participating in my study (Carpenter 2002) arose from the perceived narrow choice or lack of appropriate standardized outcome

measures in rehabilitation. This comment reflects the problem they identified:

'I really agree with the idea of objective measures, with objective outcomes appropriate for the client, but if they haven't been thought out for that individual then it's a waste of time. It's a waste of time saying I will use the Functional Independence Measure (FIM) or the Chedoke–McMaster Stroke Assessment as an objective measure of a client's improvement or function because it's generally not appropriate for that person's circumstances.'

The participants were concerned that the 'research tail was wagging the dog' – meaning that researchers, in their opinion, were unduly influenced by the availability of certain standardized instruments or that research questions were being shaped by the feasibility of implementing a desired research design. In their view, this encouraged the use of standardized outcome measurement tools that lacked the sensitivity needed to capture a client's level of function accurately. One participant's concerns are illustrated in this comment:

'The items on the Barthel Index are too gross but it is used extensively just because it has been standardized and fits experimental criteria. However, in this particular study the findings suggested that patients reached a plateau at a certain stage post-stroke but they reach a plateau because the tool couldn't register the changes that were occurring.'

The participants contrasted the relative ease of measuring the effect of specific interventions aimed at treating an acute orthopaedic problem, such as tennis elbow, with the less clearcut longer-term outcomes of interventions for people who have sustained a brain injury. This comparison is symptomatic of the fundamental difference between acute and rehabilitation care. In acute care, there is more likely to be a linear, causal, relationship between an intervention and an outcome. In contrast, rehabilitation interventions are designed with the client's larger context and goals in mind, and in collaboration with other disciplines. Rehabilitation outcomes, particularly given the decreased client admission time in centres and programmes, may be achieved only in the client's own environment after discharge from rehabilitation. The question therefore needs to be asked 'whether the purpose of judging "successful" outcomes by measuring specific [therapist identified] skills is simply a means to justify and validate current rehabilitation practice and interventions' (Hammell 2001, p. 230).

Jette & Keysor (2002) reflect these concerns in their discussion of disability outcomes and effectiveness research. Disability outcomes can be viewed 'as narrowly as the products of rehabilitation and as broadly as outcomes influenced by factors outside rehabilitation, such as the role of environmental factors in participation in life activities' (p. 327). In reality, the majority of disability outcomes and effectiveness studies continue to be dominated by descriptive epidemiological methods (Dijkers 1999, Jette & Keysor 2002). Such studies provide information for clinicians about the natural history, prevalence and/or incidence and risk factors of disease or injury, and comparative evaluations of treatments, diagnostic or other management approaches (Jette & Keysor 2002). However, they have little *direct* impact on health policies and practices, and bear little or no relationship to individual client values or preferences.

Rehabilitation practitioners consistently consider the broader 'real life outcomes of rehabilitation but not necessarily with a full awareness of the priorities of their clients' (Dijkers 1999, p. 298). Jette & Keysor (2002) suggest that a thorough discussion is needed of the relevant outcomes to pursue in rehabilitation and disability research. This discussion 'should involve not only researchers from the disability outcomes research community but also persons with disabilities, who have a unique and essential perspective on which outcomes are most relevant' (pp. 328–329). After such a determination, the research community could define and assess each outcome. Outcomes such as disability and impairment assessment, independent living, functional performance and quality of life are commonly discussed in the rehabilitation or health services literature. However, there is a lack of conceptual agreement about what is precisely meant by these or similar terms (Dijkers 1999). Recent research (Day & Jankey 1996, Woodend et al 1997) suggests that disabled people may perceive health status and quality of life differently from clinicians and researchers, and makes explicit that a broader definition of evidence is needed in

rehabilitation both to support client values, goals and preferences, and to ensure the relevance of professional programmes and services.

Establishing the efficacy of interventions or approaches to treatment has limited applicability to the reality of clinical practice in rehabilitation. Evidence of efficacy is derived from well designed studies that seek to administer the intervention in conditions deemed to be as *ideal* as possible. Effectiveness, on the other hand, is about ensuring that clinical interventions are based on the best available evidence *and* about applying such interventions within real-life conditions (Domholdt 2000). These conditions include such factors as the client's preferences and goals, client health status and characteristics, organizational systems and interdisciplinary involvement. Another way of describing clinical effectiveness was suggested by Graham (cited by Bury & Mead 1998, p. 27) as the *right* person, doing the *right* thing, the *right* way, in the *right* place, at the *right* time, with the *right* result. However, this 'six Rs' approach to clinical effectiveness continues to negate the role and preferences of the client. The current focus of evidence-based practice on outcomes and effectiveness research informs the choices of health professionals and organizations, provides accountability and improves care from a management perspective but leaves many voices unheard and questions unanswered (Miller & Crabtree 2000).

Client-centred evidence-based practice

The physiotherapists who participated in my doctoral study (Carpenter 2002) were concerned that 'best evidence' generated from quantitative research that was designed and implemented by professionals both obscured the non-quantifiable elements of clinical practice and addressed questions raised by them and not by the clients. In their view, evidence-based practice, based on a hierarchy of 'acceptable' experimental research, effectively silences the client's voice, and they regarded this as antithetical to the client-centred model of practice promoted in rehabilitation. One participant said:

'I think we have to be careful, before we go looking to see if our therapy can produce some change. We need to identify what is important or valued by patients with spinal cord injury or acquired brain injury. I mean, we've really never found out. I think that would be interesting and useful to guide our treatments.'

In physiotherapy there has been little discussion of the concept of client-centred practice, with the exception of paediatric rehabilitation where the family-centred model of care guides practice. In contrast, the client-centred model of practice has been a component of the occupational therapy philosophy since the early 1980s (Law & Mills 1998). There are a number of assumptions, according to McColl et al (1997, p. 512), associated with the client-centred approach (Box 1.2).

In summary, client-centred rehabilitation is 'a therapeutic orientation whereby clients engage the assistance and support of a therapist to facilitate their problem solving and the achievement of their own goals' (McColl et al 1997, p. 511).

Although individual professionals may strive to be client centred and health organizations may incorporate this rhetoric into their mission statements, the concept has not been consistently defined or operationalized. Significant structural changes in the organization of health care and professional education, not yet achieved, are needed to accommodate this shift in ideology from the biomedical approach (McColl et al 1997, Townsend 1998). The client-centred ethic rarely seems to influence decisions concerning what research is undertaken and how it is undertaken, or what counts as evidence for practice (Hammell 2001). In addition, few researchers have sought to

explore the meaning of client-centred practice to clients (Hammell 2001) or to ensure that the evidence accumulated is congruent with client priorities. As Corring (1999, p. 8) observed:

'Items such as the preferred approach to service delivery, priorities of treatment goals, and definitions of "rehabilitation" and "getting better" are but a few of the examples of the discrepancies between the two groups [clients and practitioners].'

In reality, evidence to support service planning, policy development and resource allocation in health care is rarely derived from experimental research or systematic reviews (Bury & Mead 1998). These decisions are multifactorial and need to be made by weighing the best possible evidence about effectiveness, cost and human resource implications, as well as local clinical experience and the views of stakeholders. More recently the client or consumer perspective and experience are being recognized as an integral and important component of these decisions (Gray 1997). Government policies are responding to consumer demands for healthcare services that are accountable, responsive to the needs of users and appropriate to individual circumstances (Department of Health 1997). These social and political pressures are reflected in the competency profile statements of both professions (e.g. Canadian Alliance of Physiotherapy Regulators et al 1998, College of Occupational Therapists 2000). There is clearly an increasing imperative to incorporate the client's values, priorities, experience and knowledge into decision-making at all levels of health care.

DIMENSIONS OF EVIDENCE-BASED PRACTICE

Evidence-based practice involves incorporating three dimensions – the conscientious and judicious use of relevant and current research evidence, clinical expertise, and patient's values and preferences – into clinical decision-making (Sackett et al 2000).

Relevant and current research

The centrality and importance of the 'best' available evidence has been discussed in detail in

---

Box 1.2 Underlying assumptions of client-centred practice

- Clients know what they need to attain their goals of care or therapy.
- The client establishes the agenda for care.
- The only relevant viewpoint or frame of reference is that of the client.
- The dominance of professionals in the therapeutic process is in fact counter-therapeutic.
- Health professionals cannot actually effect change or new learning on the part of a client; they can only create an environment that facilitates change by providing information, ideas, suggestions and resources and by establishing a relationship of trust with clients.

this chapter. However, rehabilitation practitioners are all too aware that scientific evidence is just one piece of the practice puzzle. It is simplistic to imagine that integrating the best available research evidence into practice constitutes evidence-based practice. Evidence does not make the everyday decisions in the clinical context; rather, they are made as clinicians seek to meet individual client goals. This clinical reasoning utilizes a wide range of information sources of which 'best' evidence derived from research is just one (because even 'best' evidence can lead to bad practice if applied unthinkingly or uncritically). 'The craft of caring for patients can flourish not merely in the gray zones where scientific evidence is incomplete or conflicting but also in recognition that what is black and white in the abstract may rapidly become gray when faced with the realities of clinical practice' (Naylor 1995, p. 841). Clearly, clinical practice demands the 'conscientious and *judicious* use' of research evidence, not its uncritical application. However, rigorous investigation of clinical expertise and client knowledge has evidently been subsumed by the acquisition of 'objective' evidence.

Clinical expertise

Clinical expertise represents a complex integration of theoretical knowledge, clinical reasoning and judgement, reflection on practice and skill acquisition with a patient-centred focus (Higgs & Bithell 2001). Interpretations of expertise are deeply embedded in the ways the rehabilitation professions are conceptualized, practised and managed, but are difficult to articulate and teach. *Expertise* embodies 'practice' knowledge but has been traditionally underresearched and poorly articulated (Bithell 2000, Higgs & Bithell 2001). This may explain why 'expertise' has been assigned the lowest rung of the evidentiary ladder (see Table 1.1) in comparison to 'scientific' knowledge and empirical evidence (Tonelli 1998).

Similarly, the role of theory in guiding clinical practice and research inquiry, and thus informing how rehabilitation professionals respond to individual client circumstances, has rarely been made explicit. As Banja (1997) pointed out, the rehabilitation professions have unfortunately subjected relatively few of their theories to rigorous research. This in turn provides an unstable basis for their claims to knowledge and an inadequate foundation for intervention (Hammell 2003). It is also apparent that the more powerful a professional theory becomes and the greater its longevity, the greater its ability to survive contact with contesting evidence (Childs & Williams 1997).

Client knowledge

The other dimension identified by Sackett et al (2000) is 'patient values and preferences', or client knowledge. Client-centred practice requires that clients are involved in all aspects of service provision and delivery, and that their experience and knowledge be recognized (Canadian Association of Occupational Therapists 1997). The clinical reasoning process is dependent upon solicitation of and respect for clients' knowledge, and consideration of their values and priorities, and the meaning (consequences) of disability or illness within the context of their individual lives. Such a process is compatible with a client-centred philosophy. If the elements of clinical expertise and client values, experience *and* knowledge are to be fully realized as viable sources of evidence, a shift away from a strictly positivist position is required. There is a need to rediscover the evidence missed by these research approaches – the individual and group experience and contexts, the nature of clinical expertise, 'the richness and depth of what "effectiveness" means and the human implications of rationing and cost issues' (Miller & Crabtree 2000, p. 610). Greater methodological diversity involving the use of systematic and rigorous qualitative research and multiple research paradigms gives clinical researchers the opportunity to explore more thoroughly the complexities of clinical practice and to expand the research agenda to incorporate fully clients' knowledge.

QUALITATIVE RESEARCH

Evidence generated from *quantitative* research has without question contributed to the standards and accountability of rehabilitation practice. However, the uncritical adoption of this research paradigm has limited our ability to investigate the complexities of clinical practice and 'practice' knowledge, to engage in collaborative research projects with other health professional or consumer groups, or to capitalize on clients' knowledge or understand their perspectives. The desire to capture the individual's point of view, examine the constraints of everyday life and secure rich descriptions of the social world (Denzin & Lincoln 2000) can be addressed more effectively by *qualitative* research.

Qualitative research is sometimes presented as 'a basket of technical tools, devoid of epistemological and theoretical basis that underpin its claims to be a legitimate means of generating knowledge' (Popay & Williams 1998, p. 35). Most committed qualitative researchers would contest this simplistic interpretation as they struggle with such terms as paradigm, theory, epistemology, interpretive framework, methodology and methods, in their attempts to define qualitative research clearly. Qualitative research, according to Denzin & Lincoln (2000), is a 'set of interpretive activities' that has 'no theory or paradigm that is distinctly its own', nor does it 'privilege a single methodology over another' (p. 6). It draws upon and utilizes a diversity of approaches, methods and techniques, such as ethnography, phenomenology, feminism, hermeneutics and grounded theory. As a result, qualitative research is difficult to define. Qualitative researchers do, however, share a similar world view. Qualitative researchers 'approach the world with a set of ideas and values, a framework (theory, ontology) that specifies a set of questions (epistemology) that he or she then examines in specific ways (methodology, analysis)' (Denzin & Lincoln 2000, p. 18). The net that contains the researcher's epistemological, ontological and methodological premises may be termed a paradigm or interpretive framework, a basic set of beliefs and ideas (Lincoln & Guba 2000). All research, including the positivist paradigm, is interpretive; it is guided by a set of beliefs and feelings about the world (ontology) and how it should be understood and studied, that is, how knowledge should be generated (epistemology). 'Each interpretive paradigm makes particular demands on the researcher,

including the questions he or she asks and the interpretations the researcher brings to them' (Denzin & Lincoln 2000, p. 19). From an ontological standpoint, qualitative researchers believe that there is no single 'reality' to be discovered. Rather, there are multiple constructed realities to be understood. Qualitative research is based on an interpretive epistemology, meaning that knowledge is generated and shaped through interaction between those involved in the research process. Qualitative methodologies are concerned with how the researcher can explore and analyse whatever it is he or she believes can be known, and are based upon prior epistemological assumptions (Hammell 2002).

There is some confusion in the health research literature regarding the terms 'methodology' and 'method', and often they are mistakenly used interchangeably. *Methodology* refers to a theory of how knowledge can be developed and how research ought to proceed given the nature of the issue it seeks to address. It is thus a philosophical consideration. Research *methods* are techniques and strategies employed to acquire knowledge and manipulate data, consistent with the chosen methodology (Hammell & Carpenter 2000). In qualitative research such methods as individual, in-depth interviewing, participant observation and focus groups are commonly used.

In summary, different qualitative research approaches can share certain assumptions or characteristics (Hammell & Carpenter 2000) and these are outlined in Box 1.3.

Qualitative research approaches acknowledge 'the value-laden nature of inquiry, and seek meaning and understanding ahead of quantifiable measures. They deal with the socially constructed nature of reality, the close relationship [between participants and researcher], and the frequent necessity to investigate without stripping the phenomenon under study of its context' (Ritchie 2001, p. 150).

THE CONTRIBUTION OF QUALITATIVE EVIDENCE

Proponents of evidence-based practice have traditionally emphasized quantitative methods and

Box 1.3 Shared assumptions and characteristics of qualitative enquiry

- Research is grounded in people's everyday lives and in an exploration of how people experience and make sense of dimensions (e.g. interventions, events, relationships) of their lives.
- Human behaviour can only be understood in context.
- People, including the researcher, perceive and interpret reality differently; there are multiple realities rather than an 'objective' truth to be discovered.
- Research is conducted in a 'natural' setting (as opposed to controlled or laboratory settings).
- The research process is initiated by 'problems' or 'irritants' arising from the experience of everyday life or the 'realities' of clinical practice.
- The researcher is an integral part of the research process. The issue is not one of minimizing the researcher's role but of describing and explaining it thoroughly.
- Data analysis is inductive and interpretive.
- Data are presented in narrative form with the aim of preserving and representing the participants' voices.

subsequently placed high value on numerical data. Increasingly, it is being recognized that such data 'may in reality be misleading, reductionist, and irrelevant to the real issues' (Greenhalgh 1997, p. 743). As Miller & Crabtree (2000) suggest: 'the new gold standard, if there should be any at all, needs to include qualitative methods along with the randomised controlled trial' (p. 613). In health care there is a marked difference or gap between seeking an objective research outcome and pursuing an individual clinical care outcome, and it would appear that 'the error lies in the narrow definition of the term evidence' (Ritchie 2001, p. 173). Bridging this gap is the role of qualitative research. It is becoming imperative that the definition of evidence be broadened through the inclusion of qualitative methods if all the dimensions are to be brought into focus in the total picture of evidence-based practice.

This book is premised on our conviction that rigorous and systematic qualitative research can potentially be used to address complex rehabilitation practice issues, justify decisions and explore issues in service provision and resource allocation, facilitate examination and development of theory, and illuminate clinical expertise. The

occupational therapy profession has engaged in explicit discussions of their theoretical underpinnings. However, according to De Souza (1998), complex physical therapy practice is rather like 'a black box', the contents of which are tacitly understood and applied by therapists. However, what guides their judgements is not clear. Qualitative research helps 'to surface hidden theoretical assumptions and suggest new possibilities and connections' (Miller & Crabtree 2000, p. 615) and can be used to reaffirm, revise or expand an existing theoretical framework (Hammell & Carpenter 2000). Philosophically compatible with a client-centred ethic, qualitative methods enable researchers to identify ways in which therapy interventions and modes of service delivery may be better crafted to meet the needs and priorities of clients. 'There has been little research into the individual clinical expertise side of the evidence-based equation and the associated areas of relationship dynamics, communication, and patient preference, and there is much to be learned about how clients and clinicians implement "best evidence"' (Miller & Crabtree 2000, p. 613). In addition, the emphasis on quantitative research has focused attention on causal relationships, on the products or outcomes of interventions, and on *how* to effect the desired results – and less on *why* things happen the way they do. The *why* entails a broader understanding of the system of wide-ranging theories or ideas that therapists hold about their practice, and their interaction with clients and other professionals.

Qualitative research addresses questions not readily answered by quantitative methods. Popay & Williams (1998) identified a number of ways in which qualitative research can contribute to evidence-based practice. These included: challenging taken-for-granted practices; illuminating factors that shape client and clinical behaviour; developing new interventions based on clients' experiences; evaluating and determining optimal outcomes of care; enhancing understanding of organizational culture and the management of change; and evaluating service delivery. Increasingly, qualitative findings are being reported in the literature and are contributing unique evidence upon which to base rehabilitation practice.

Two examples of qualitative studies illustrate this kind of contribution. Cook & Hassenkamp (2000) identified the need, in evaluating active rehabilitation programmes for clients with chronic low back pain, to establish that such programmes were meeting the clients' needs as well as demonstrating significant objective outcomes. The findings indicated that outcomes were influenced as much by the clients' perceptions of health and quality of life, the group culture and dynamics of the treatment programme, and clients' experiences in their own environments as by physiotherapy interventions. They recommended that combining qualitative research with controlled trials offered a more effective approach to addressing the wide-ranging issues surrounding the management of these problems. Segal (1998) identified that, although families as the main caregivers of children with special needs are a primary focus of client-centred occupational therapy practice, no research involving families with children who have attention deficit/hyperactivity disorder (ADHD) had been reported in the occupational therapy literature. Her qualitative study reported the interaction between enabling strategies developed by the parents and the daily routines of family members. The study findings contribute to occupational therapists' ability to develop cooperative partnerships with families caring for children who have ADHD and to provide relevant and effective services for them. Other examples of studies that have contributed in these ways are provided in the ensuing chapters of this book.

EVIDENCE-BASED REHABILITATION: INFORMING PRACTICE THROUGH QUALITATIVE RESEARCH

The aim of this book is to address the role of qualitative research in enhancing both the theoretical and knowledge bases of occupational therapy and physiotherapy that inform evidence-based practice. To achieve that aim, we invited researchers from both professions to discuss the evidence generated from specific examples of qualitative research studies. The resulting chapters illustrate the contribution that qualitative methods can

make in a number of areas: theory development and application, understanding clients' health-related perceptions, exploring professional practice and clinical expertise, evaluation of service delivery in the community, and the use of multiple research methods.

In Chapter 2, Karen Whalley Hammell uses qualitative research into the everyday lives of people with high spinal cord injuries living in the community to critique and develop theories of occupation. In Chapter 3, Melinda Suto bases her discussion of the theoretical development of leisure on her research, in which she uses an ethnographic approach to explore how resettlement shapes the definition, meaning and role that leisure plays in the lives of women who immigrate to Canada. In Chapter 4, Mary Law describes how a participatory research study was used to explore disabling environments that affect the daily occupations of children with disabilities and how this qualitative evidence can be used to inform practice and theory development. In Chapter 5, I discuss how qualitative evidence derived from a participatory research study evaluating the role of an advocacy organization and the programmes it provides for clients living with spinal cord injury can make an important contribution to service evaluation and delivery. In Chapter 6, Deborah Corring describes her research journey using a participatory action approach to explore how clients with mental illness define client-centred care and quality of life, and discusses the impact of this important information on rehabilitation practice. In Chapter 7, Candice Schachter and colleagues describe their research collaboration with women survivors of childhood sexual abuse in exploring their reactions to physical therapy and the subsequent development of principles of sensitive practice for clinicians. In Chapter 8, Karen Rebeiro describes a series of participatory action research studies that led to the development of a collaborative, occupation-based mental health initiative. In Chapter 9, Jan Gwyer and colleagues highlight the findings of qualitative research that used a multiple case study approach, and how these findings lead to an enhanced understanding of clinical expertise in physical therapy and the development of a theoretical model of expert practice for the profession. In Chapter 10, Michael Curtin and Emily Jaramazovic demonstrate how their use of mixed qualitative and quantitative methods in exploring occupational therapists' perceptions of evidence-based practice can enhance both practice standards and the relevance of quantitative research.

The studies described and the issues raised in these chapters illustrate the complex and multi-faceted nature of the questions addressed by qualitative research, and the richness and depth of evidence that such research can generate. The value of qualitative research is dependent on researchers' commitment to ensuring the transparency of the research process and thus the rigour and trustworthiness of the research. Acquiring this kind of evidence will require qualitative researchers to develop cross-disciplinary collaborations, to combine research methodologies and use multiple research methods, and to emphasize participatory and advocacy approaches (Miller & Crabtree 2000). In the concluding chapter, Karen Whalley Hammell will draw on the preceding chapters in reviewing some of the many ways in which the evidence derived from qualitative research can be used to inform practice, and sketch some additional methods of qualitative research not addressed in previous chapters. She will conclude by reviewing some suggested guidelines for critical appraisal of qualitative studies and examine the potential and possibilities for mixing qualitative research methods with those of quantitative research.

REFERENCES

Banja JD 1997 Values and outcomes: the ethical implications of multiple meanings. Topics in Stroke Rehabilitation 4(2):59–70

Baum C, Christiansen C 1997 The occupational therapy context: philosophy – principles – practice. In: Christiansen C, Baum C (eds) Occupational therapy: enabling, function and well-being. 2nd edn. Slack, Thorofare, NJ; pp. 26–45

Bithell C 2000 Evidence-based physiotherapy: some thoughts on 'best evidence'. Physiotherapy 86(2):58–61

Bury TJ, Mead JM 1998 Evidence-based healthcare explained. In: Bury TJ, Mead JM (eds) Evidence-based healthcare: a practical guide for therapists. Butterworth Heinemann, Oxford; pp. 4–25

Canadian Alliance of Physiotherapy Regulators, Canadian Physiotherapy Association, Canadian University Physical Therapy Academic Council 1998 Competency profile for the entry-level physiotherapist in Canada. Canadian Physiotherapy Association, Toronto

Canadian Association of Occupational Therapists 1997 Enabling occupation. An occupational therapy perspective. CAOT, Ottawa

Canadian Association of Occupational Therapists, Association of Canadian Occupational Therapy University Programs, Association of Canadian Occupational Therapy Regulatory Organizations, Presidents' Advisory Committee 1999 Joint position statement on evidence-based occupational therapy. Canadian Journal of Occupational Therapy 66(5):267–279

Carpenter C 2002 Dilemmas of practice in rehabilitation settings as experienced by physical therapists. PhD thesis, University of British Columbia, Vancouver

Carse A, Nelson H 1996 Rehabilitating care. Kennedy Institute of Ethics Journal 6(1):19–35

Childs P, Williams P 1997 An introduction to post-colonial theory. Prentice-Hall, London

College of Occupational Therapists 2000 Code of ethics and professional conduct for occupational therapists. College of Occupational Therapists, London

Cook FM, Hassenkamp A-M 2000 Active rehabilitation for chronic low back pain: the patients' perspective. Physiotherapy 86(2):61–68

Corring D 1999 The missing perspective on client-centered care. OT Now Jan–Feb:8–10

Council of Directors of Physical Therapy Academic Programs, Canadian Physiotherapy Association 1995 Entry-level curriculum for Canadian physical therapy programs: guidelines for faculty. Canadian Physiotherapy Association, Toronto

Day H, Jankey SG 1996 Lessons from the literature: toward a model of quality of life. In: Renwick R, Brown I, Nagler M (eds) Quality of life in health promotion and rehabilitation. Sage, Thousand Oaks, CA; pp. 39–50

Denzin N, Lincoln Y (eds) 2000 Introduction: the discipline and practice of qualitative research. In: Handbook of qualitative research. 2nd edn. Sage, Thousand Oaks, CA; pp. 1–29

Department of Health 1997 Policy research programme: providing a knowledge base for health, public health and social care. Department of Health, London

De Souza L 1998 Theories about therapies are underdeveloped (editorial). Physiotherapy Research International 3(3):iv–vi

Dijkers M 1999 Measuring quality of life: methodological issues. American Journal of Physical Medicine and Rehabilitation 78(3):286–300

Domholdt E 2000 Physical therapy research: principles and applications. 2nd edn. WB Saunders, Philadelphia

Evidence-Based Working Group 1992 Evidence-based medicine. Journal of the American Medical Association 268:2420–2425

Finch E, Brooks D, Stratford P 2002 Physical therapy rehabilitation outcome measures. 2nd edn. Canadian Physiotherapy Association, Toronto

Gray J 1997 Evidence-based healthcare: how to make health policy and management decisions. Churchill Livingstone, Edinburgh

Greenhalgh T 1997 Assessing the methodological quality of published papers. British Medical Journal 315:305–308

Hammell KW 2001 Using qualitative research to inform the client-centered evidence-based practice of occupational therapy. British Journal of Occupational Therapy 64(5):228–234

Hammell KW 2002 Informing client-centred practice through qualitative enquiry: evaluating the quality of qualitative research. British Journal of Occupational Therapy 65(4):175–184

Hammell KW 2003 The rehabilitation process. In: Stokes M, Ashburn A (eds) Physical management in neurological rehabilitation. 2nd edn. Harcourt, Edinburgh

Hammell KW, Carpenter C 2000 Introduction to qualitative research in occupational therapy and physical therapy. In: Hammell KW, Carpenter C, Dyck I (eds) Using qualitative research: a practical introduction for occupational and physical therapists. Churchill Livingstone, Edinburgh; pp. 1–12

Herbert R, Sherrington C, Maher C, Moseley A 2001 Evidence-based practice – imperfect but necessary. Physiotherapy Theory and Practice 17:201–211

Higgs J, Bithell C 2001 Professional expertise. In: Higgs J, Titchen A (eds) Practice knowledge and expertise in the health professions. Butterworth-Heinemann, Oxford; pp. 59–68

Jette A, Keysor J 2002 Uses of evidence in disability outcomes and effectiveness research. The Milbank Quarterly 80(2):325–345

Law M (ed) 1998 Client-centered occupational therapy. Slack, Thorofare, NJ

Law M (ed) 2002 Evidence-based rehabilitation: a guide to practice. Slack, Thorofare, NJ

Law M, Mills J 1998 Client-centered occupational therapy. In: Law M (ed) Client-centered occupational therapy. Slack, Thorofare, NJ; pp. 1–18

Lincoln Y, Guba E 2000 Paradigmatic controversies, contradictions, and emerging confluences. In: Denzin N, Lincoln Y (eds) Handbook of qualitative research. 2nd edn. Sage, Thousand Oaks, CA; pp. 163–188

Maynard A 1997 Evidence-based medicine: an incomplete method for informing treatment choices. Lancet 349:126–128

McColl M, Gerein N, Valentine F 1997 Meeting the challenges of disability. Models for enabling function and well-being. In: Christiansen C, Baum C (eds) Occupational therapy: enabling function and well-being. 2nd edn. Slack, Thorofare, NJ; pp. 509–528

Miller W, Crabtree B 2000 Clinical research. In: Denzin N, Lincoln Y (eds) Handbook of qualitative research. 2nd edn. Sage, Thousand Oaks, CA; pp. 607–631

Naylor CD 1995 Grey zones of clinical practice: some limits to evidence-based medicine. Lancet 345:840–842

Nicholson D 2002 Practice guidelines, algorithms, and clinical pathways. In: Law M (ed) Evidence-based rehabilitation: a guide to practice. Slack, Thorofare, NJ; pp. 195–220

Popay J, Williams G 1998 Qualitative research and evidence-based healthcare. Journal of the Royal Society of Medicine 91(suppl 35):32–37

Ritchie J 2001 Not everything can be reduced to numbers. In: Berglund C (ed) Health Research. Oxford University Press, Oxford; pp. 149–173

Rosenberg W, Donald A 1995 Evidence-based medicine: an approach to clinical problem-solving. British Medical Journal 3(10):1122–1126

Roskell C, Hewison A, Wildman S 1998 The theory–practice gap and physiotherapy in the UK: insights from the nursing experience. Physiotherapy Theory and Practice 14:223–233

Sackett D, Richardson W, Rosenberg W, Haynes R 1996 Evidence-based medicine. Churchill Livingstone, Edinburgh

Sackett D, Strauss S, Richardson W, Rosenberg W, Haynes R 2000 Evidence-based medicine. How to practice and teach EBM. 2nd edn. Churchill Livingstone, Edinburgh

Segal R 1998 The construction of family occupations: a study of families with children who have attention deficit/hyperactivity disorder. Canadian Journal of Occupational Therapy 65(5):286–292

Sumsion T 1997 Client-centered implications of evidence-based practice. Physiotherapy 83(7):373–378

Tanenbaum S 1999 Evidence and expertise: the challenge of the outcomes movement to medical professionalism. Academic Medicine 74(7):757–763

Taylor MC 2000 Evidence-based practice for occupational therapy. Blackwell, Oxford

Tonelli MR 1998 The philosophical limits of evidence-based medicine. Academic Medicine 73(12):1234–1240

Townsend E 1998 Good intentions overruled: a critique of empowerment in the routine organization of mental health services. University of Toronto, Toronto

Townsend E, Rebeiro K 2001 Canada's joint position statement on evidence-based occupational therapy. OT Now Jan/Feb:8–11

Woodend AK, Nair RC, Tang AS 1997 Definition of life quality from a patient perspective versus health care professional perspective. International Journal of Rehabilitation Research 20:71–80

FURTHER READING

Hammell KW, Carpenter C, Dyck I 2000 (eds) Using qualitative research: a practical introduction for occupational and physical therapists. Churchill Livingstone, Edinburgh

Morse JM, Swanson JM, Kuzer AJ 2001 The nature of qualitative evidence. Sage, Thousand Oaks, CA

2

Using qualitative evidence to inform theories of occupation

Karen Whalley Hammell

KEY POINTS
relating qualitative research findings to theory; theories of occupation; client-centred research; high spinal cord injury (C1–C4)

OVERVIEW

The next three chapters discuss the generation of theory from qualitative research evidence. Theory informs what we believe should be done in various situations, thus sound clinical practice demands a strong theoretical base. Evidence-based practice supports the importance of establishing interventions that are informed by dependable theory. Claims to dependability require that theories are firmly grounded in research evidence. In this chapter, Karen Whalley Hammell demonstrates how evidence derived from qualitative research can be used to inform the theoretical underpinnings of occupational therapy, enabling clients' perspectives to infiltrate theory. Arguing that client-centred practice must be informed by theories derived from clients' perspectives, she illustrates how client-generated perspectives may contest and challenge the normative, ableist assumptions of theorists and therapists.

INTRODUCTION

This chapter uses qualitative research into the everyday lives of people with high spinal cord injuries to critique and develop theories of occupation. *Occupation* is central to the conceptual foundation of occupational therapy, yet despite the profession's declared allegiance to client-centredness there has been little effort to include the perspectives of diverse client groups in the development of theories of occupation. This chapter demonstrates how qualitative methodology may provide a client-centred approach to theory building, critiquing the assumptions that underlie the shared beliefs of the profession and exposing for debate the values that underpin them.

INTRODUCING THE RESEARCH: EXPLORING QUALITY IN LIFE FOLLOWING HIGH SPINAL CORD INJURY

This interdisciplinary study was designed to explore perceptions of 'quality in life' (the experience of a life worth living) among men and women with high traumatic tetraplegia (quadriplegia) and the factors they identified as contributing to, enabling or constraining, their lives.

What prompted the research?

Review of the research literature demonstrated that little effort had been expended to determine whether people who are completely paralysed below the neck following high spinal cord injuries feel satisfied with their lives or perceive survival to be worthwhile. In light of evidence that healthcare providers believe death to be preferable to life with this injury (Gerhart 1997), and because scant information was available on which to ground relevant and useful rehabilitation services for these survivors, it appeared important to understand more about the lives that are being saved in increasing numbers. I was persuaded that seeking to comprehend whether a meaningful life is possible following such profound injury and determining *what kind* of life is possible would provide useful insights to inform future clinical decision-making, rehabilitation programmes and social policies. My assumption appeared to be supported by comments from the participants, such as: 'This is really important work you're doing'.

Fitting the research methodology and methods to the research purpose

A qualitative methodology was chosen to explore the experience of living with high spinal cord injury because in the absence of previous research the study would be exploratory, because a qualitative methodology is appropriate to examine issues that are, by definition, concerned with quality and not quantity (e.g. quality of life), and because it was congruent with the expressed wish of some participants to explain their lives 'in our own voices' (Hammell 2000, p. 60).

THE RESEARCH PROCESS
Study participants

Men and women were invited to participate in the study if they had complete, traumatic spinal cord injuries between C1 and C4, were at least 2 years' postinjury, aged between 20 and 50 years, and living in the community in the Lower Mainland of British Columbia or on Vancouver Island. These criteria were selected to enable consideration of the impact of gender on the experience of disability (which would be precluded if only one gender was selected for study), to consider the experience of people in a relatively homogeneous age group (and one most commonly affected by spinal cord injury) who had attained some lengthy experience living with this injury, and to enable access for me, as the researcher. Potential participants were identified by a method of 'snowball sampling' (Bogdan & Biklen 1998), whereby some participants suggested the names of others they knew who would meet the stated criteria (see Hammell 2000).

Everyone who was invited to participate agreed to do so, representing probably every person in this geographical area who met the inclusion criteria (and therefore precluding the possibility of sample bias). Participants were both men (11) and women (4), of mixed ethnicity, and who therefore provided a degree of triangulation by informant diversity. *Triangulation* is a strategy to enhance the trustworthiness of research and is based on the premise that comparison of perspectives enables corroboration, illumination or elaboration of the data (Marshall & Rossman 1989). Age at injury ranged from 12 to 44 years, with a mode of 24 years. The number of years since injury varied from 4 to 28 years.

Ethics and consent

Approval for the study was granted by the Behavioral Research Ethics Board of the University of British Columbia. After reading the informed consent form, each person was offered the choice of signing consent (by holding a pen between their teeth) or stating verbal consent directly on to the audio tape.

Data collection: methods, process, documentation

Semi-structured interviews were selected to explore the experience of living with complete paralysis below the neck from the perspectives of people with high tetraplegia (for more details see Hammell 2000). Semi-structured interviews enable insight into the logic by which participants interpret their lives and permit a glimpse into their life worlds and daily experiences (McCracken 1988). Each interview was guided by a basic checklist of issues that enabled every person to address the same topics. The interviews were initially informed by my knowledge of both high tetraplegia and the academic and disability literatures, and subsequently informed by the issues raised by the participants so that data collection and analysis were intermeshed (see Hammell 2000). After interviewing each person, second interviews were undertaken with the first five people I had met, enabling me to explore further some of the issues that had been raised during the course of the study.

All except one of the interviews were audiotaped and subsequently transcribed verbatim (one person preferred not to have a recording made). This eliminated the need to take notes during the interviews and enabled me to capture and preserve the conversations in their entirety for subsequent in-depth analysis.

Field notes were recorded immediately after each interview as a means to document perceptions and impressions of the interview and the dynamics of our interaction (Carpenter & Hammell 2000). A diary was used to record any problems, discrepancies or gaps in the information being generated and any ideas or hypotheses that arose. The diary therefore provided a forum for reflection and identification of emergent themes.

During the course of the interviews I became a transient but active participant in the lives of the study participants. I answered their telephones, wiped away tears, moved arms and legs, performed assisted coughs, passed cups, positioned drinking straws and provided whatever additional information I was asked for, whether this pertained, for example, to wheelchair cushions, feminism and disability, or the state of 'cure' research. Reciprocity and attempts to minimize power imbalances are characteristics of qualitative research methodology (Oakley 1981).

In an attempt to reflect occupational therapy's client-centred philosophy and to respond to the demands of disability activists for accountable and collaborative research, concerted efforts were made to involve participants throughout the research process (see Hammell 2000). This 'member checking' (Krefting 1991) assured a degree of triangulation by incorporating a diversity of perspectives throughout the research process (Hammell 2002). Any discrepancies that arose prompted further reflection and renewed efforts to understand and privilege the participants' perspectives.

The study was conducted over a period of several months until I was satisfied that the data had become 'saturated' (Bogdan & Biklen 1998), that is, no new themes were emerging – new stories confirmed what was already understood while adding only slight individual variations – and when I had confirmed or explicated these themes through repeat interviews.

Reflexivity and the researcher role

Reflexivity refers to the conscious examination of the position of the researcher within the research. It is recognized that the biographical 'position' – gender, ethnicity, class, 'race', sexual orientation, age, religion, (dis)ability, professional status, education and other dimensions of social differentiation – of the researcher will affect the research relationship and the nature of the data collected (Carpenter & Hammell 2000). Likewise, the researcher's philosophical positioning affects the degree to which power is shared within the research process and the degree of accountability to the participant group that the researcher strives to achieve (Hammell 2000). Respect for the principle of client-centredness and a desire to ensure the relevance and value of the research to the community I had elected to study informed my own approach to this process.

My stated familiarity with high spinal cord injury (as a result of my husband's injury) and desire to capture the perspectives of the 'insiders' on a topic that was important to the participants appeared to guarantee the participation in the project of all those who were invited. More importantly, it may have contributed to the depth of our conversations and encouraged them to recruit my assistance with various personal tasks. As one young man observed: 'I'm glad to see somebody like you doing something like this'.

Power relations in the research process

Disability theorists have drawn attention to the power imbalances between those who research and those who are researched (Oliver 1997). Traditional modes of research in which the researcher controls the research design, how the study is conducted, analysed, written up and disseminated sit uncomfortably with client-centred philosophy (Hammell 2002). It is not possible to erase power differentials but attempts were made to contest them in this study, for example by involving participants in developing the research issues and discussing my interpretations of the data, engaging in interactive interviews (including answering questions and providing information) and acquiescing to participants' suggestions for the dissemination of research findings (Hammell 2000, 2002).

Data analysis and theoretical constructs

Through a process of writing a line by line index of the transcribed interviews, summarizing these by words or phrases, and creating a visual 'tally' of the themes that arose during the interviews, I identified 'coding categories' (Bogdan & Biklen 1998) that accounted for all the data (excluding only data that pertained to specific individuals, such as the experience of cocaine addiction). These coding categories were clearly defined on index cards and the cards were then arranged thematically, such that related issues were included within one theme. Thus, categories that had resonance with other similar categories were related within one theme. Once this thematic analysis of the data had been undertaken, the findings were related to contemporary theories and the interpretations were discussed with a key participant in an effort to ensure both plausibility and authenticity (Hammell 2000). *Plausibility* is concerned with ensuring that the findings of a study 'fit' the data from which they are derived (Sandelowski 1986). *Authenticity* pertains to the reliability and trustworthiness of the research process (Carpenter & Hammell 2000).

Respondent validation

In an attempt to reflect occupational therapy's espoused commitment to client-centredness, participant involvement was sought throughout the research process. Respondent validation ('member checking') included, for example, incorporating participants' perspectives into data analysis by asking some participants to clarify interpretations and to review and comment on the categories and themes that I was identifying in the data. I also endeavoured to ensure that participants were comfortable with how their experiences were to be used and guaranteed access to the findings for the peer groups from which the study participants were drawn (Hammell 2002). The first papers that I wrote concerning the research were therefore submitted to publications produced by and for disabled people and suggested by the study participants (Hammell 2000).

THE RESEARCH FINDINGS

It was apparent that high spinal cord injury had disrupted not just a body but an entire biography of plans, daily activities and valued occupations. Initially feeling helpless and useless, life itself had held little value and assisted suicide, for some, appeared a seductive option. However, the participants were unanimously glad to be alive at the time of the study and several reported lives that were more focused, less superficial and more meaningful and rewarding than prior to injury (Hammell 1998). The themes that emerged from the data were overlapping and interdependent, and described a process of re-establishing a view of the self as able and valuable following injury. These themes appear in Box 2.1.

Autonomy

The opportunity to be in control of one's own life was strongly linked to perceptions of quality in

> **Box 2.1** Emerging themes
>
> - Autonomy, choice and control; and the related issue of deinstitutionalization
> - Meaningful use of time
> - Relationships.

living. Ability was discerned not by how many activities the participants could accomplish without assistance but by how much control they had over their lives. This sense of autonomy was set in opposition to the experience of institutionalization.

Several participants described the restricted and impoverished environment of the institutions in which they had resided for many years. They described feelings of imprisonment, helplessness, dependency and occupational deprivation. They explained that they had been unable to contribute to others, participate in society or enact adult roles. Several people stated that death would be favoured over a return to living in a long-term care facility. Some of the study participants had been instrumental in forcing innovative changes in social policy that have enabled them to hire their own assistants and live where and with whom they choose. The success of this model of care enabled others to follow, so all the participants in this study lived in the community with support from paid assistants, sometimes supplemented by help from parents or spouses.

Meaningful use of time

The importance of doing

Sudden confrontation with the fragility of life had forced a revision of the values that informed the use of time. Engaging in meaningful activities was shown to fill life with purpose and imbue it with quality: 'You can do a lot, and *make* a quality of life' (David). The participants emphasized the importance of 'doing something', and included five elements within this theme. These themes are outlined in Box 2.2, illustrated by participants' comments (all names are pseudonyms to preserve anonymity). The ability to determine daily activities contributed to a sense of autonomy, and was thus linked to the previous theme.

Box 2.2 The importance of doing

- The need to keep busy:

'I think probably when I first got hurt, I felt my life was over, but once you get on with things and get doing different things, you know it's not by any means ... I have to be doing something' (Eric). 'I just like to keep busy' (Ingrid). 'I keep really busy ... you just find some sort of challenge and it really keeps you occupied ... It's about what we can DO' (David). 'I need to be busy' (Katherine).

- The need to have something to wake up for:

'Painting is something to look forward to – something to do when I get up' (Colin). '[after a while] you realize that you've got options and you've got something that you can wake up for every day – I've got to DO something today ... We all need something to wake up for' (David).

- The chance to explore new opportunities:

'I do different kinds of things like short stories, poetry ... writing kind of replaced the hole when I couldn't play music anymore ... and it is something I feel really proud of ... I'd never tried writing until after my

accident. It was something totally new that I didn't know I had' (Luke). 'A lot of doors have opened for me that probably never would have! I know I would never have painted and I REALLY enjoy that. I know that I would have never met some people that I have' (David).

- The need to envisage future time engaged in valued activities:

'I'm going for my dreams and goals – and that's school and getting a good education to have a good job ... It gives me encouragement that I'm doing something good with my life' (Ingrid). 'You've got the rest of your life in front of you ... you can't spend a lot of time worrying about what you can't do. Figure out what you can do and focus on that' (Erik).

- The need to contribute reciprocally to others:

'We need to be able to contribute. We need to be able to give back' (Alan). 'I'm a kind of counsellor ... I have a lot of people who come to me with problems, so ... I feel I can contribute' (Matthew). 'I'm able to contribute ... I can do things that will make a difference for other people with disabilities' (Beth).

The importance of being

The participants also stressed the importance of time spent in contemplation and in appreciation of the 'taken for granted' – such as sunshine, a shower, or being alone, counterbalancing society's emphasis on 'busy-ness' with a state of introspection and passive enjoyment that I termed 'being'. For example, since his injury Nicholas has rejected his former lifestyle of material comforts and social prestige, viewing it as shallow and superficial. He pursues university studies in philosophy, values time spent in quiet contemplation and the opportunity to 'sit in solitude – enjoy the fresh air'.

Owen described the factors that contribute to his pleasure in life, to making life worth living:

'I think it's mostly just watching the kids. Things that other people [take for granted] – I don't take for granted any more. And the best thing is I can look out of the back window here and watch the birds and watch the wind blow in the wind sock or the trees around ... just watching pretty simple things ... I think I've got a bit of an edge over most people that are working all the time because I get to watch my [children] grow up'.

Relationships

This theme picks up on the idea of contributing to others that was seen in the context of time use. The participants emphasized the importance of those relationships characterized by reciprocity and mutual support. Relationships with special people contributed to the experience of life's quality and also comprised an important resource in reconstructing a life worth living.

While relationships with family members, friends, intimates and assistants affirmed the worth and value of the injured person, their practical and emotional support had enabled the exploration and exploitation of life opportunities. As David explained:

'[my family] didn't treat me any differently, they just sort of said, "Well, this has happened, now how do we get around it? How do we make the most of it?"'

Study conclusions

Since leaving institutional custody the participants' lives have come to resemble those of other members of society. Several have married, some have fathered children, some have attained university degrees or are currently studying for academic or professional qualifications. Some are employed, full-time, others volunteer or pursue artistic, literary or business endeavours. Once the participants were able to regain control of their everyday lives, they redefined themselves as able, capable and valuable. Indeed, many no longer viewed themselves as 'disabled'.

The findings from this research suggest that quality of life outcomes might be maximized by adopting two approaches. First, because the onset of high spinal cord injury is not solely an assault on a physical body but on a life, a biographical orientation to rehabilitation would help to ensure that interventions are meaningful, useful and relevant to the individual in the context of their environment, and are focused on fostering control and a view of the self as able and competent.

It is also apparent that a focus upon modifying individuals may be less important than efforts to modify environments. Quality in living for this group of people had been enabled by social policy initiatives including: universal health care, direct funding for personal assistants, accessible public transportation and housing; provision of high-technology equipment and sip-and-puff power wheelchairs, access to education and employment options and financial support. Pre-occupation with individual dysfunction is clearly an insufficient response to the circumstances of high tetraplegia.

In conclusion, the research demonstrated that life with a high spinal cord injury could be rich and fulfilling if society was prepared to enable and support this.

RELATING CURRENT FINDINGS TO EXISTING THEORY

Many qualitative researchers advocate for an intellectually engaged form of analysis that moves beyond simply identifying and describing themes within individual studies (unfortunately still a common practice in occupational therapy research), to discussing the meaning of the data, exploring how study findings relate to, contest or further existing theories (e.g. Frank 1997, Hammell 2002, Lyons et al 2002, Secker et al 1995).

'Theory, although understated (or even unstated) is what guides all clinical practice and every research inquiry: informing what we believe should be done in various situations' (Hammell & Carpenter 2000, p. 10). Evidence-based practice supports the importance of establishing interventions that are informed by dependable theory. Because client-centredness has become an ethical requirement for occupational therapy practice, the research base that informs client-centred theory and practice should reflect a client-centred orientation. 'Clearly, the philosophy underpinning the development of the evidence base destined to provide guidelines for practice should be ethically consistent with the espoused practice philosophy' (Hammell 2001, p. 229). Qualitative methods enable researchers to study phenomena from the perspectives of the participants and to explore the meanings with which they make sense of their lives and experiences, thus increasing the chance that theories emerging from qualitative research will be relevant (Hammell & Carpenter 2000). Qualitative data can be used to reaffirm, revise or expand a particular theoretical framework, expose limits to current theories, and identify previously unrecognized relationships among elements of a phenomenon (Hammell 2001, Hammell & Carpenter 2000). Thematic analysis of data from this research study demonstrated its fit with theories of occupation.

Occupation: defining the term

As an occupational therapist, I approached this study into the experience of high spinal cord injury informed by a literature base that claimed the centrality of occupation to the experience of being human but which had few research studies to support this premise. Indeed, while study of *occupation* would seem to be central to the discipline of occupational therapy, there is no consensus on the precise definition of this word. Seeking to avoid value-laden descriptors, I choose to define occupation as anything that people do in their daily lives (McColl et al 1992).

Occupational therapists hold several assumptions concerning occupation. These include (Canadian Association of Occupational Therapists 1997, Yerxa et al 1989):

- occupation is a determinant of health
- occupation is a source of meaning
- occupation is a source of purpose
- occupation is a source of choice and control
- occupation is a source of balance
- occupation is a means to express and manage identity
- occupations are chunks of activities
- occupations may be classified into self-care, productive or leisure activities.

Occupation as a determinant of health

Occupational therapy is grounded in the premise that engagement in occupations influences health (Yerxa et al 1989). This study challenged a traditional assumption of the link between occupation and health. It suggested that occupations do not need to be physically undertaken by an individual in order to contribute to a positive sense of well-being. David, for example, described building a patio – directing his staff to build a patio – and of his enjoyment and sense of accomplishment in planning and undertaking this project. There can be a 'virtual' link between occupation and well-being (health) that is not directly attributed to physiology or physical function.

Occupation as a source of meaning and purpose

It was evident that the study participants identified the importance of engagement in both purposeful and personally meaningful occupations. Occupation is defined by several influential writers solely in terms of purpose. For example, occupations are said to be 'all purposeful human activity' (Wilcock 1998a, p. 22) and have also been described as 'self-initiated, goal-directed (purposeful), and socially sanctioned' activities (Yerxa et al 1989, p. 5). I term this *doing*. In contrast, several of the participants in this study described an enjoyment of time that

I termed *being*, which comprised dimensions of time use that are not captured by classificatory systems devised by able-bodied, career-oriented academics, for whom self-initiated, goal-directed, socially sanctioned activities reflect specific priorities and values.

Some writers define occupations as personally meaningful activities but then proceed to discuss purposeful activities, suggesting that they perceive the words purposeful and meaningful to be somehow interchangeable. For example, Fougeyrollas (1998, p. 145) defines occupation both as 'any meaningful activity or task in which humans engage as part of their normal daily lives' (citing McColl et al 1992) and 'in short' as 'goal-oriented use of time' (citing Christiansen & Baum 1997). I contend that these two definitions are neither compatible nor interchangeable (although the first may include the second as a subset) and cannot be collapsed into one concept. The Canadian Association of Occupational Therapists (CAOT 1997, p. 36) states that 'Meaning differs from purpose in occupation'; thus occupations can be meaningful without having any identifiable purpose.

By describing rewarding use of time engaged in occupations that I termed 'being', the study participants challenged the normative judgement that values only 'purposeful' occupations. Several people described a richly satisfying use of time that reflected personal values, thereby suggesting that occupations do not need to be purposeful to be contributors to quality in living.

Mee & Sumsion (2001) suggested that doing something purposeful is directly associated with the meaning of one's day and that engagement in occupations that are personally meaningful contributes to a sense of purpose. However, it would appear spurious to interchange the words such that meaningful becomes a pseudonym for purposeful.

It is stated that: 'Occupations are meaningful to people when they fulfil a goal or purpose that is personally or culturally important' (CAOT 1997, p. 36). Use of the word meaningful in this context implies that this is a positive term, yet all occupations are meaningful: they all have some meaning for the individual engaged in them. The meaning with which an activity is imbued may be positive or negative, and may change by time and context. Rejecting the suggestion that 'meaningful occupations' are those that are 'chosen and performed to generate experiences of personal meaning' (CAOT 1997, p. 181), I propose instead that *all* occupations are endowed with meaning and that the experience of engagement in occupations will be dependent upon the meaning or interpretation with which the occupation is imbued. It may therefore be more precise to refer to 'personally meaningful' occupations when wishing to denote activities that are valued by the individual.

Occupation as a source of choice and control

Previous researchers have reported that perceptions of being in control of one's life are positively associated with the experience of quality in life (e.g. Fuhrer et al 1992). These findings were strongly supported by the participants in this study, who demonstrated that the process of refocusing their lives entailed a reassertion of authorship over everyday life activities and reaffirmation of competency. They justified Yerxa et al's (1989) premise that 'to engage in occupations is to *take control*' (p. 5).

People can express choice and exercise control in their lives when they have opportunities to decide what they will do (CAOT 1997). Importantly, 'control is more than choice. People may make choices about their occupations but have little control to act on choices' (CAOT 1997, p. 37). This was evident from the participants' experiences of institutionalization.

There is an apparent linkage between the right to autonomy and ability to enact choices concerning the meaningful use of time (both highly valued by the participants), and human rights. The research indicates the need to draw upon a wide range of services and supports in the process of engaging in chosen occupations. These included (but were not limited to) personal assistants, accessible transportation, financial supports, education and employment opportunities, and deinstitutionalization, supporting the premise that 'Control is dependent on opportunities provided by the environment' (CAOT 1997, p. 37).

Occupation as a source of balance

'One of the most widely cited philosophical beliefs in occupational therapy is that a balance of occupations is beneficial to health and well-being' (Christiansen 1996, p. 432). However, Clark et al (1991, p. 306) observe that, while this assumption may be valid, it 'fails to define work, leisure, or what constitutes a balance; does not specify the aspects of health that are promoted; and is not seriously subjected to the possibility of disconfirmation'. The study participants were unanimous in describing the time-filling self-care demands of life with a severe impairment and the consequent limit on time available for engagement in personally meaningful occupations that would balance their physical care needs with time spent in ways deemed valuable and rewarding. Hagedorn (1995) proposed that the concept of balance among occupations 'does not relate to work, leisure and self-care, but to a harmony between utility and meaning in the life of the individual' (p. 149). This conceptualization of balance most neatly encapsulates this study's findings.

Occupation as a means to express and manage identity

Vrkljan & Miller-Polgar (2001) suggest a connection between engagement in meaningful occupations and self-perceptions of being a capable person that reflect the findings of this study. When someone sustains a spinal cord injury, 'it is not just that the person can no longer walk, it is that the actions of life that were enjoyably self-defining are no longer available' (Lee et al 1993, pp. 205–206). When the study participants lost their ability to do the activities that were important to them, this negatively impacted their perceptions of themselves as capable and they described feeling useless and valueless. Conversely, when they resumed participation in valued occupations, they redefined themselves as valuable and capable rather than disabled. Luke described the benefits he derives from writing and studying:

'I think it gives me an identity … I remember when I was always really concerned how my girlfriend would introduce me to her friends, 'cause I just didn't want to be known as the boyfriend in a wheelchair 'cause it's a total stigma ... and I asked her about it and she said, "Well, I just introduce you as my boyfriend and you're just a student and a writer, you know, and the wheelchair part never comes up".'

The able self was depicted as the occupational self.

Occupations as chunks of activity

Occupations have been defined as 'chunks' of daily activity that can be named in the lexicon of the culture (Yerxa et al 1989). The idea that people engage in only one sort of activity at any given moment in time also informs the use of activity diaries in which research participants are instructed to note the activities in which they are engaged at certain periods of the day.

This study into life with high tetraplegia suggests that this notion of 'chunking' represents an ableist perspective on daily life: the assumption that one can accomplish one activity at a time and then get on with something else. (*Ableism* refers to social relations and practices that assume and privilege able-bodiedness.) For most able-bodied academics who develop these theories, self-care activities, for example, probably can be performed in chunks of time. For people with high tetraplegia the need to protect the skin, suction the lungs, avoid overheating or cooling, and drink substantial volumes of water mean that measures to maintain the body are interwoven with every other activity. Beth, for example, was describing her efforts to maintain her human rights within the confines of an institution when she suddenly asked me to check whether her arm was lying against my tape recorder (and thereby susceptible to skin damage). When I visited Heather, a small alarm rang at regular intervals to remind her to alter the angle of tilt of her wheelchair and thus the pressure on her skin and underlying tissues. I suggest that the onset of severe impairment demands conscious attention to self-care on a continual basis such that these activities are integral to all others and cannot be neatly segregated or 'chunked'.

Classifying occupations

Occupational therapists tend to divide occupations into categories of self-care, productivity and leisure (CAOT 1997). However, several researchers have identified problems with classifying activities. Not only may the same activity be defined as productive by some people and as leisure by others, but the same individual may define the same activity differently at different times (CAOT 1997), reinforcing the premise that meaningful occupations do not generate consistent experiences of meaning. Time of day, mood, location of activity and the presence of other people may all affect the definition and meaning attributed to any given activity at any moment in time.

The findings of this study challenge the premise that occupations can be neatly delineated or categorized (as indicated in the section on 'chunking'). The demands of the tetraplegic body mean that self-care activities protrude into every other activity such that occupations are always multilayered rather than divided into identifiable chunks. This contributes to the difficulty of chunking and classifying occupations, and thereafter determining what constitutes 'balance' between them.

Several previous studies have found social activity to be positively associated with life satisfaction (e.g. Fuhrer et al 1992, Krause 1991). In this study, I was unable to differentiate the notion of 'social activity' from the dual concepts of relationships and doing. When the study participants spoke of their relationships with family and friends, it was frequently in the context of activities such as going to restaurants, bars, theatres or concerts. Similarly, important relationships often underpinned the ability to 'do', for example travelling and pursuing higher education, suggesting that the satisfaction associated with relationships and occupational engagement cannot be simplistically labelled 'leisure', 'productive' or 'social'. Rather, relationships both contributed to the pleasure of 'doing' and underpinned the ability 'to do'. This adds to the difficulties in defining and categorizing occupations.

It is evident that listing occupations as self-care, productive or leisure (e.g. CAOT 1997) is neither a random nor an alphabetical ordering. Rather, this reflects the values and priorities of theorists (see Ch. 3). Devault (1990) observes that naming activities is not a neutral act but value-laden and inherently political: 'the labels attached to activities establish and justify their social worth' (p. 110).

Some disability theorists would contend that by prioritizing self-care and productive (especially income-generating) activities, occupational therapists act as agents of the state, actively perpetuating political ideologies that reinforce inequality and marginalize those deemed 'dependent' and 'unproductive'. By perpetuating ideals of superiority and inferiority, dominant cultural values can be oppressive to disabled people who may be unable – or unwilling – to conform to ableism's ideals.

Occupations that defy definition

While it was apparent that some activities might be classified into several categories – for example, use of the telephone may be for leisure and socializing, part of a productive work activity or a dimension of self-care in arranging personal assistants' schedules – others defy definition.

Christopher Reeve described his experience of returning to his rural home for the first time since his high spinal cord injury: 'I parked myself on a ramp. It was a beautiful, cool afternoon, and I just looked up at the mountains for about two hours and felt very, very peaceful' (Time 1996, p. 47). Clearly this was an experience that held a great deal of personal meaning, but which was neither productive nor leisure, and fits more closely the theme identified as 'being'. This again raises issues regarding occupational therapy's espoused priority on 'purposeful' occupations.

Rowles (1991) observed that a predominant focus on doing 'has tended to overshadow *being* as an essential ingredient of human experience' (p. 265). Rowles proposed that 'to live as a fully self-actualizing person involves the process of being, of simply experiencing life and the environment around us, frequently in an accepting, non-instrumental way. Being, in this sense, involves the realms of meaning, value, and intentionality that imbue our lives with a richness and diversity that transcends what we know and what we do' (p. 265). Priority on 'doing' is not a universal cultural value.

Occupation: doing, being and becoming

Wilcock (1998b) observed that, while some theorists see occupation as comprised of goal-directed, purposeful activities, occupation 'is more than "doing". It is a synthesis of doing, being and becoming' (p. 341).

Frank (1995, p. 159) suggested that after the initial shock of a diagnosis has dulled somewhat, the individual must surely consider, 'What do you wish to *become* in this experience? What story do you wish to tell of yourself?'. Kleiber et al (1995) proposed that 'the new story one writes for oneself subsequent to traumatic life events … is quite likely to be illustrated with a future self in action in a way that makes life enjoyable and meaningful once again' (p. 297).

The importance of occupation was identified as integral to the process of refocusing lives disrupted by spinal cord injury, restoring valued self-identities, and using time in ways perceived to be meaningful and fulfilling. I suggest that engagement in occupation contributes to a sense of 'becoming': becoming capable, becoming valuable and creating a life worth living.

CONCLUDING THOUGHTS

The theoretical basis for occupational therapy has been generated primarily without client input. Sound clinical practice demands a strong theoretical basis, but theory developed in the absence of clients' perspectives provides an unstable basis from which to inform client-centred practice. This chapter has demonstrated how evidence derived from qualitative research might inform the theoretical knowledge base of occupational therapy, enabling client-generated perspectives to infiltrate theory.

Occupational therapy is premised on the belief that engagement in occupation gives meaning to life (Yerxa et al 1989). While strongly supporting this theory, the participants provided further insights that could usefully inform theories of occupation (Box 2.3).

Few previous studies have explored engagement in daily occupations following spinal cord injury. However, research has indicated that people who are more active in social and productive occupations are more likely to survive following their spinal cord injuries (e.g. Krause 1991). This suggests that engagement in personally meaningful occupations may not only have a role in

Box 2.3 Building theory from clients' perspectives

- Directing others in purposeful occupations contributes positively to well-being.
- Engaging in purposeful occupations contributes to meaning and quality in living.
- Engaging in personally meaningful occupations contributes to quality in living.
- To be personally meaningful, occupations do not need to be purposeful.
- Environmental factors may enable or constrain autonomy and occupational choice.
- Balance of occupations refers to a harmony between utility and personal meaning.
- Occupation is a means to express identity and achieve a sense of competence and value.
- Occupations cannot be segregated into chunks.
- Occupations cannot be classified according to their apparent characteristics.
- Current systems of classification are value-laden, reflecting the priorities of theorists and therapists.
- Some occupations cannot be made to fit into existing frameworks of classification.
- Occupations may comprise elements of doing and being in a process of becoming: pursuing a life that is personally meaningful and imbued with quality.

reconstructing self-identity and in using time in a fulfilling manner following injury, but occupation may also influence survival itself.

ACKNOWLEDGEMENTS

I am greatly indebted to the 15 people with high lesion tetraplegia, their families and assistants, who welcomed both me and my study. The research upon which this chapter is based was generously supported by the following: University of British Columbia Graduate Fellowship, Rick Hansen Man in Motion Foundation Studentship, Social Sciences and Humanities Research Council of Canada Doctoral Fellowship.

REFERENCES

Bogdan RC, Biklen SK 1998 Qualitative research for education. An introduction to theory and methods. 3rd edn. Allyn & Bacon, Boston

Canadian Association of Occupational Therapists 1997 Enabling occupation. An occupational therapy perspective. CAOT, Ottawa

Carpenter C, Hammell KW 2000 Evaluating qualitative research. In: Hammell KW, Carpenter C, Dyck I (eds) Using qualitative research: a practical introduction for occupational and physical therapists. Harcourt, Oxford; pp. 107–119

Christiansen CH 1996 Three perspectives on balance in occupation. In: Zemke R, Clark F (eds) Occupational science: the evolving discipline. FA Davis, Philadelphia; pp. 431–451

Christiansen C, Baum C 1997 Occupational therapy: enhancing human performance. Slack, Thorofare, NJ

Clark F, Parham D, Carlson M et al 1991 Occupational science: academic innovation in the service of occupational therapy's future. American Journal of Occupational Therapy 45(4):300–310

Devault ML 1990 Talking and listening from women's standpoint: feminist strategies for interviewing and analysis. Social Problems 31(1):96–116

Fougeyrollas P 1998 Consequences for occupation. In: McColl MA, Bickenbach JE (eds) Introduction to disability. WB Saunders, London; pp. 145–150

Frank AW 1995 The wounded storyteller. Body, illness and ethics. University of Chicago Press, Chicago

Frank G 1997 Is there life after categories? Reflexivity in qualitative research. Occupational Therapy Journal of Research 17(2):84–98

Fuhrer MJ, Rintala DH, Hart KA et al 1992 Relationship of life satisfaction to impairment, disability and handicap among persons with spinal cord injury living in the community. Archives of Physical Medicine and Rehabilitation 73:552–557

Gerhart KA 1997 Quality of life: the danger of differing perceptions. Topics in Spinal Cord Injury Rehabilitation 2(3):78–84

Hagedorn R 1995 Occupational therapy. Perspectives and processes. Churchill Livingstone, Edinburgh

Hammell KW 1998 From the neck up: quality in life following high spinal cord injury. Doctoral thesis, University of British Columbia, Vancouver

Hammell KW 2000 Representation and accountability in qualitative research. In: Hammell KW, Carpenter C, Dyck I (eds) Using qualitative research: a practical introduction for occupational and physical therapists. Harcourt, Oxford; pp. 59–71

Hammell KW 2001 Using qualitative research to inform the client-centred evidence-based practice of occupational therapy. British Journal of Occupational Therapy 64(5):228–234

Hammell KW 2002 Informing client-centred practice through qualitative inquiry: evaluating the quality of qualitative research. British Journal of Occupational Therapy 65(4):175–184

Hammell KW, Carpenter C 2000 Introduction to qualitative research in occupational and physical therapy. In: Hammell KW, Carpenter C, Dyck I (eds) Using qualitative research: a practical introduction for occupational and physical therapists. Harcourt, Oxford; pp. 1–12

Kleiber DA, Brock SC, Lee Y et al 1995 The relevance of leisure in an illness experience: realities of spinal cord injury. Journal of Leisure Research 27(3):283–299

Krause JS 1991 Survival following spinal cord injury: a fifteen-year prospective study. Rehabilitation Psychology 36(2):89–98

Krefting L 1991 Rigor in qualitative research: the assessment of trustworthiness. American Journal of Occupational Therapy 45(3):214–222

Lee Y, Brock S, Datillo J et al 1993 Leisure and adjustment to spinal cord injury: conceptual and methodological suggestions. Therapeutic Recreation Journal Third quarter:200–211

Lyons M, Orozovic N, Davis J, Newman J 2002 Doing–being–becoming: occupational experiences of persons with life-threatening illnesses. American Journal of Occupational Therapy 56:285–295

Marshall C, Rossman GB 1989 Designing qualitative research. Sage, Newbury Park, CA

McColl MA, Law M, Stewart D 1992 Theoretical basis of occupational therapy. Slack, Thorofare, NJ

McCracken G 1988 The long interview. Sage, Newbury Park, CA

Mee J, Sumsion T 2001 Mental health clients confirm the motivating power of occupation. British Journal of Occupational Therapy 64(3):121–128

Oakley A 1981 Interviewing women: a contradiction in terms. In: Roberts H (ed) Doing feminist research. Routledge, London; pp. 30–61

Oliver M 1997 Emancipatory research: realistic goal or impossible dream? In: Barnes C, Mercer G (eds) Doing disability research. The Disability Press, Leeds; pp. 15–31

Rowles GD 1991 Beyond performance: being in place as a component of occupational therapy. American Journal of Occupational Therapy 45(3):265–271

Sandelowski M 1986 The problem of rigor in qualitative research. Advances in Nursing Science 8(3):27–37

Secker J, Wimbush E, Watson J, Milburn K 1995 Qualitative methods in health promotion research: some criteria for quality. Health Education Journal 54:74–87

Time 1996 New hopes, new dreams. Time 26 August:36–48

Vrkljan B, Miller-Polgar J 2001 Meaning of occupational engagement in life-threatening illness: a qualitative pilot project. Canadian Journal of Occupational Therapy 68(4):237–246

Wilcock AA 1998a An occupational perspective of health. Slack, Thorofare, NJ

Wilcock AA 1998b Reflections on doing, being and becoming. Canadian Journal of Occupational Therapy 65(5):248–256

Yerxa EJ, Clark F, Frank G et al 1989 An introduction to occupational science: a foundation for occupational therapy in the 21st century. Occupational Therapy in Health Care 6(5):1–17

FURTHER READING

Barton L 1996 Disability and society: emerging issues and insights. Longman, London

Carpenter C 1994 The experience of spinal cord injury: the individual's perspective – implications for rehabilitation practice. Physical Therapy 74(7):614–629

Kirsch GE 1999 Ethical dilemmas in feminist research. The politics of location, interpretation and publication. State University of New York Press, Albany, NY

Lyons M, Orozovic N, Davis J, Newman J 2002 Doing–being–becoming: occupational experiences of persons with life-threatening illnesses. American Journal of Occupational Therapy 56:285–295

3

Exploring leisure meanings that inform client-centred practice

Melinda Suto

KEY POINTS

Canadian Model of Occupational Performance; environment; gender, race and class; women and resettlement; evidence for rethinking leisure in context; leisure as a dimension of life; using qualitative evidence to inform theory

OVERVIEW

Melinda Suto's chapter continues the exploration of ways in which the evidence derived from qualitative research can be used to critique and develop theory. Noting the centrality of leisure within theories of occupation, yet the curious dearth of supportive research evidence, Melinda's research sought to explore how gender, 'race' and class function to shape the meaning and experience of leisure. By enabling actual and potential clients to contribute to the development of theory, her research reflected occupational therapy's espoused commitment to client-centredness and empowerment. Melinda argues in this chapter: 'While practice provides the litmus test for concepts and theories, research is necessary to clarify concepts, ensure their rigorous examination, and confirm their basis in research evidence'.

K.H.

INTRODUCTION

This chapter addresses the lack of conceptual development regarding leisure in occupational therapy models and the implications for practice that this situation creates. A critical theory perspective is taken to examine assumptions and omissions of leisure within the Canadian Model of Occupational Performance, which presents itself as client-centred and inclusive (Canadian Association of Occupational Therapists (CAOT) 1997). The research design and question challenge occupational therapy's pragmatic approach to leisure. Using an ethnographic approach and semi-structured interviews, I address the question of how resettlement shapes the definition, meaning and role that leisure plays in the lives of women who immigrate to Canada. The different experiences of 'leisure' for women who immigrate to Canada are examined through the trifocal lens of gender, race and class relations. The findings provide evidence for leisure as a dimension of life, embedded within family and community social life. Revealing the multiple meanings attributed to 'leisure' activities and the importance of context demonstrates the role of qualitative methodology in furthering the theoretical development of leisure to enable client-centred practice.

THE PROBLEM OF LEISURE IN OCCUPATIONAL THERAPY

Leisure and the quest for balance

The centrality of leisure in occupational therapy conceptual models demands a rigorous examination of the concept (CAOT 1997, Kielhofner 1995). However, the conceptual development of leisure in

occupational therapy is rudimentary. Since the profession began in the early twentieth century, leisure participation has been associated uncritically with good health and a balanced life (Knox 1998). The inclusion of leisure as a necessary ingredient for a balanced life may be explained partly by 'class' values and opportunities. The profession's founders in the United States were positioned firmly in the upper-middle class (Frank 1992). Unlike the working-class people they primarily treated, early occupational therapy practitioners had a social orientation to leisure and the financial means to access it. Contemporary analyses of leisure from within occupational therapy remain curiously absent in the literature. Primeau's (1996) examination of work and leisure in relation to a balanced life stands as a notable exception.

Traditionally, occupational therapy has sought concepts outside the profession, customizing them for practice and research purposes. If occupational therapy continues to import concepts from other disciplines, it must critically examine the usefulness of these concepts. The pertinent questions for leisure in occupational therapy are legion, for example: How does occupational therapy define leisure? What scholarly literature and perspectives provide the evidence for this definition and understanding of leisure? Do practitioners expect that all of their clients share this prevailing view of leisure? How do the social relations of daily life shape clients' understanding of leisure and participation in it? To understand whether leisure is part of a balanced life, what constitutes 'balance' and what people from diverse backgrounds understand as leisure, we need answers to some of these questions. As an academic working in Canada, the main occupational therapy practice model used in Canada is the logical place to begin the search.

Canadian Model of Occupational Performance

Assumptions and omissions

The Canadian Model of Occupational Performance (CAOT 1997) describes an environment with social, cultural, institutional and physical elements that shape occupation. The model proposes that the outcome of interaction between environment, occupation and person produces occupational performance. Occupation is divided into three areas: self-care, productivity and leisure. The belief that occupation comprises these areas, and the typical placement of leisure last, reflect occupational therapy's value-laden assumptions and priorities. As an occupational performance area, leisure is supported by practice based in tradition. While practice provides the litmus test for concepts and theories, research is necessary to clarify concepts, ensure their rigorous examination, and confirm their basis in research evidence.

In *Enabling Occupation* (CAOT 1997), gender, race and class are mentioned in the context of questions of discrimination that need to be studied using critical social science analyses. How the authors theorize these concepts is not addressed. Neither are the authors' own gender, race and class subject to critical analysis – nor the impact of their positioning on their theoretical perspectives. A critical examination of how these social relations influence the meanings of leisure is absent in this book. Given the position of the environment in the model – but perhaps consistent with the suggestion that occupational therapists focus predominantly on the physical environment – this omission is surprising. My approach to gender, race and class theorizes these as social relations that shape everyday experiences, including leisure. Their linkage together implies that no one concept is privileged over another. Consistent with Ng's (1998) use of these concepts, race, class and gender are understood to overlap, functioning as dynamic forces. As interactive processes, these social relations offer people opportunities to contest representations of themselves by society. The use of this trio of concepts in this research is 'for discovering how they are relations that organize our productive and reproductive activities, which are located in time and space' (Ng 1998, p. 22). The research discussed here addresses the knowledge gap regarding how leisure fits into the larger context of our clients' lives. Simply put, there are two problems: we know little about leisure and even less about how gender, race and class function to shape the meaning and experience of leisure.

Implications of omitting a critical analysis of leisure

The absence of leisure from occupational therapy's conceptual map has implications for students, therapists and clients. Occupational therapy educators who wish to present leisure in a more nuanced way have few resources. Thus leisure is presented to students uncritically: as tangible activities or as a domain of a client's life. Through observation as students, and later as practitioners, occupational therapists begin to grasp whether and how leisure functions in their clients' lives. This inadvertent devaluation of leisure as worthy of serious study has the potential to compromise rehabilitation. First, it encourages occupational therapists to rely primarily on understandings of leisure from popular culture and their own experiences. The life circumstances that enable these experiences may be different from those of their clients. Second, occupational therapists risk remaining focused at the individual level. A lack of awareness about the larger social forces that shape clients' lives can disadvantage the practice of an otherwise excellent occupational therapist. Third, assessments of clients' leisure preferences presume implicit understandings of and access to leisure. Fourth, conceptual lack of clarity concerning leisure serves to devalue it, redirecting the focus towards the more tangible areas of self-care and productivity, that is, leading to a neglect of an area that we claim to be essential for 'balance'. These unstated assumptions may impede strategies to incorporate leisure into targeted outcomes of therapy.

The impetus for this research arises from the conceptual status of leisure in occupational therapy. This research also recognizes the postmodern shift to challenging professional dominance over the development of knowledge and fostering empowerment (CAOT 1997).

Empowerment through research

Empowerment is linked inextricably to occupational therapy theory and practice. It is claimed to be an outcome of the enablement process, which is itself an essential feature of occupational therapy.

Yet, while client-centredness and empowerment are core values of practice and are central to theory, these are not characteristics of theory development or research. In Canadian occupational therapy, empowerment is defined as 'personal and social processes that transform visible and invisible relationships so that power is shared more equally' (CAOT 1997, p. 180). Involving people other than occupational therapists in leisure research can identify assumptions of practice, allow the profession to question the validity of its beliefs, and enable actual and potential clients to contribute to the development of theory. For example, there is an implicit assumption that leisure is a relevant concept to most, if not all, occupational therapy clients. Individual practitioners work collaboratively to understand the role that leisure plays in their clients' lives, but seldom is that role questioned. I want this research to challenge how occupational therapists think about leisure. I chose to listen to the voices of people who are not typically consulted in the development of theory: women who immigrate to Canada and reconstruct their lives here.

Leisure: a dimension of life

The assumption that leisure is a unique occupational performance area, rather than a dimension of life, is uncontested in occupational therapy. This research examines how leisure is defined and, in doing so, begins to challenge the status of leisure as an area of occupational performance. Three general definitions of leisure reflected in occupational therapy practice are presented, followed by a proposal for a more nuanced definition. These definitions set the stage for the research findings that argue for leisure as a dimension of life, woven into the social relations of everyday life and inseparable from those relations.

Definitions of leisure

Despite its prominence in the Canadian Model of Occupational Performance, leisure is defined simply as 'enjoying life' (CAOT 1997, p. 34). Presumably this definition arises from understanding leisure as time, activity and/or subjective experience. The notion of leisure as comprising quantifiable chunks of time is familiar to occupational therapists. We use activity configurations, time budgets, diaries, the 'pie of life' and other modalities to assess how clients use time, including leisure time. The idea of leisure as time gained prominence when the nature of work changed in response to industrialization. Social changes meant that leisure occurred outside of the work environment; it was considered the opposite of work, and the amount of time for leisure differed between men and women (Primeau 1996). Mosey defines leisure as 'time when one is free from family and other social responsibilities, activities of daily living, and work. It is characterized by a feeling of comparative freedom and self-determination' (cited in Reed & Sanderson 1999, pp. 150–151).

The notion of leisure as an activity is familiar to occupational therapists through assessments such as the Activity Checklist (Katz 1988). This checklist is used to identify activities that include leisure (tennis, chess) and would be recognizable as leisure activities by many North Americans. Other checklist items (ironing, floor mopping and mathematics) suggest the variety of activities that draw one's attention and curiosity. Indeed, these kinds of activities may even be experienced as 'leisure' sometimes, highlighting the problem of defining leisure by specific activities.

Understanding leisure as subjective experience refers to leisure as one's state of mind when engaged in occupations. These occupations may not be identifiable to outsiders as leisure activities. The advantage of this perspective is the recognition of degrees of leisure experienced within occupations rather than the occupations themselves. The experiential view of leisure encourages an examination of qualities associated with leisure, such as freedom of choice, perceived competence, flow and relaxation. To capture the importance of the meaning that clients give to leisure, I propose using the following definition (Reid 1995, p. 14):

'Leisure will be defined as those activities which produce intrinsic rewards and provide the participant with life-enhancing meaning and a sense of pleasure... What often separates work from leisure is the attitude with which it is undertaken and the reward which is gained from the experience. With work, the reward is often only monetary; leisure usually involves intrinsic value. Leisure, then, is as much an attitude or state of mind, as it is a type of activity.'

Reid's definition highlights the subjective nature of leisure, while acknowledging the activity focus. It provides a position from which to explore leisure as a dimension of life.

METHODOLOGY

Ethnographic approach

The type of question the researcher seeks to address influences the choice of methodology. The research question I posed was: 'In what ways does the process of resettlement in Canada influence the definition, meaning and role that leisure plays in women's lives?' This question arises from occupational therapy's scant knowledge of how resettlement influences the restructuring of lives in a new environment (Creese et al 1999). Thus I am interested in examining how this experience shapes the meanings women give to leisure and where leisure fits in their lives. The methodology comprises an ethnographic approach with critical theories, informed by feminism and postcolonial writing. An ethnographic approach produces an in-depth understanding of complex phenomena within particular contexts. Context refers to the micro and macro environments that influence women's resettlement experiences. The interpretations and meanings women construct around leisure in their lives are dependent on context, among other things. The emphasis on context (which is congruent with occupational therapy's environmental interest) and the contribution of critical theories differentiates the chosen methodology from other approaches, such as phenomenological or constructivist.

Critical theory

The objective of critical theory is to critique the socially constructed experiences of people, understand the nature of power relations and empower people to change their lives (Kincheloe & McLaren

1994). The diverse writings that constitute post-colonial critical theory critique the construction of the 'other' (Said 1978). The production of discourses concerning 'immigrant woman' is an example of creating the 'other'. In the Canadian context, changes to immigration policy and the emergence of state-sanctioned multiculturalism are identified as fostering this construction of difference (Ng 1998). Researchers using postcolonial critical theory analyse how particular creations of 'otherness' or difference arise. Why a construction of an 'other' emerges when it does, who benefits from it, and what impact it has on women's lives are the kinds of questions that researchers ask. Critical theorists argue that this concept of difference contributes to a process of stereotyping and racialization that immigrants from developing countries experience (Thobani 2000). Central to this analysis is how the discourse of 'immigrant woman' influences the social relations of class, gender and race that are part of everyday life. Postcolonial critical theory offers a historical and political perspective from which to analyse how power relations affect people's lives.

Feminist critical perspectives share an interest in the relations of power with postcolonial theories but focus the analytical lens on gender. By definition, feminist methodology aims to 'correct both the invisibility and distortion of female experience in ways relevant to ending women's unequal social position' (Lather 1991, p. 71). This highlights another feature of critical theory methodology: that the researcher's values be made explicit because they guide the research process. For example, critical researchers recognize that research can recreate conditions of inequality and contribute to some forms of oppression. Critical theorists strive to conduct research in ways that reduce power differentials through attention to how knowledge is created. The methods I used in this research reflect the values I place on empowerment and equality.

Methods

Semi-structured, in-depth interviews constituted the primary means of data collection in this study. This style of interview allowed me to pose similar questions to all the women who participated in the research (hereafter referred to as 'participants'). The semi-structured nature of the interviews encouraged participants to direct the conversation to topics that they thought relevant to the research questions. This is especially important in an exploratory study where the researcher does not always know the issues of concern to participants before commencing the study. It also reflects the values inherent in the methodology.

Participant observation is customary in research that uses an ethnographic approach. However, it was inappropriate for this study because the main research question concerned the meaning and role of leisure for women. Therefore, personal perspectives were of central interest rather than any actual activities.

Another method of data collection was a log of daily activities, kept over a 1- or 2-day period. The purpose of this method was to help each participant reflect on whether she engaged in leisure, the extent to which leisure might occur in her daily activities, and the experiences that were labelled as 'leisure' by the participants. Recognizing that the plausibility of the findings might be strengthened by additional data collection strategies influenced my choice of this method.

THE RESEARCH PROCESS

Recruitment

The flexible and unpredictable nature of qualitative research designs was demonstrated in the recruitment of participants. Initially I planned to recruit women from three multicultural service agencies that had offered their assistance. Despite presentations to staff working with immigrants and repeated telephone follow-up, 6 months of recruitment efforts from these agencies were unsuccessful. This situation prompted a return to the literature to determine whether changing the inclusion criteria was justified.

Theoretical sample

The original theoretical sample proposed that participants be women between 25 and 45 years old, who had lived in Canada for between 3 and 10

years having arrived after the age of 19. I sought participants who could be interviewed in English, which was necessary owing to a lack of funding for translation services. Although unstated, I had hoped to recruit women whose family income suggested the concept of 'working' class. In contrast with women whose family income is high, I reasoned that women from lower income families would be more challenged by juggling domestic responsibilities, paid work and learning English. Therefore, it seemed likely that the role that leisure may have played in their lives prior to immigration would change considerably as new priorities were established.

Because of the difficulty in attaining a participant group, the new theoretical sample that was constructed required an age range of 20–55 years and employment became an unnecessary criterion, owing to the difficulty in obtaining work. The 'middle years' of resettlement, defined in the literature as residency of between 2 and 12 years, became a target rather than a rigid criterion. This time period is thought to be one of integration to Canadian society, following the initial period of immediate adjustment (Rose et al 1998). After presenting my research plan directly to participants in two immigrant integration programmes, 13 women agreed to join the study. Seven women volunteered after hearing about the research from friends, through their own work with immigrants or via written advertisements. After further changes to the sample criteria, interviews with 13 women constituted the data (Table 3.1). Nine research participants were recruited from immigrant integration programmes and four from other sources. The reason for this reduction was to create a sample of women who shared similar demographic characteristics. The high number of participants in this study who had completed post-secondary education can be explained by two factors. First, 31% of 25–44-year-old women who immigrated between 1991 and 1996 had completed post-secondary education (Badets & Howatson-Leo 1999). Only 20% of Canadian-born women in the same age group completed this level of education. Second, being well educated increases the likelihood that women had developed some English language skills prior to entering Canada.

Table 3.1 Demographic data of the 13 participants

Pseudonym	Country of origin	Age (years)	Education	Year of arrival in Canada
Isabelle	Philippines (Manila)	43	PhD (economics) + two master's degrees	1995
Graciela	Mexico (Mexico City)	39	BA (psychology) + other courses	1998
Rosa	Guatemala (rural)	33	MS (international relations)	1991
Maira	Bosnia (Sarajevo)	37	PhD (linguistics)	1994
Fereshteh	Iran (Tehran)	50	BA (social work)	1999
Maria	Mexico (Culiacan)	30	BEd + other courses	1993
Ling	Taiwan (Taipei)	43	BA (sociology)	1998
Alicia	Mexico (Mexico City)	30	1 year of university	1998
Svetlana	Ukraine (Zaporozhye)	45	MSc (electrical engineering)	1999
Chin-sung	Taiwan (Taipei)	40	BA (business administration)	2000
Sonia	India (Uttar Pradesh)	31	BA (law)	1999
Mila	Bosnia (Sarajevo)	41	BA (architecture)	1995
Dolores	Mexico (Cordoba)	31	BA (business administration)	1999

Ethnographic interviewing

Each interview was held at a location suggested by the participant, most often in her home but occasionally in coffee shops. Informed consent forms were discussed and signed by all participants just before each interview. The interviews lasted for 1–2 hours, with the average of around 90 minutes. Each participant was interviewed once and agreed to be audiotaped. Audiotaping allowed me to focus on the content and process of the interview. This was essential because English was a second language for all of the participants and I speak only English. Some words were difficult to understand during the interview. This and the accented English spoken posed challenges to the professional transcriber I employed. She did not have access to the non-verbal communication that accompanied each interview, and which often helped me to identify the participants' words. Recognizing that words and meanings could be lost in the transcription process prompted me to repeat and paraphrase more frequently than is desirable with this type of interview. The danger in paraphrasing is that the researcher may inadvertently produce a 'mini-analysis' of the meaning of the participant's comment. This has the potential to lead the interview towards confirming the researcher's preconceived ideas rather than exploring the participant's perspective and experience. It also interrupts the flow of the interview.

Transcription of audiotapes

I shared the transcription of audiotapes with a professional transcriber. Verbatim transcription of an interview preserves the participant's words and helps the researcher remain true to the speaker's intent. The necessity of speaking in English sometimes limited the depth to which participants could discuss the meaning of leisure in their lives. The ability to describe clearly the meanings ascribed to one's actions is enhanced by an extensive vocabulary, and attempts to discuss the meanings that participants gave to leisure experiences were sometimes thwarted by a limited English vocabulary. In contrast, participants appeared to describe their daily activities with relative ease, including those activities they defined as leisure.

Interview questions

The phrasing of questions reveals some of the researcher's preconceived understanding about the topic from the literature and provides structure for the interview. The interview guide in Box 3.1 lists the main questions asked of all participants. The order and wording varied slightly and prompting questions elicited further elaboration. In these interviews, I tried to ask questions simply and briefly. Sometimes I offered participants an explanation of the concept of leisure, which may have restricted the dialogue that

Box 3.1 Interview guide

- Can you describe, in detail, your typical daily activities on a weekday?
- From what you have described, which activities would you describe as leisure?
- Can you tell me what qualities the activities have that make them leisure?
- Can you describe how important these activities are to you now?
- What does it mean to you when you cannot engage in these activities?
- Is there something you would like to do, but cannot due to other constraints?
- How do you describe leisure?
- In what ways, if at all, do you think leisure is related to a person's health?
- Can you describe how leisure fits into how you assess your own health?
- Are the resources for leisure available in your home country different from those in Canada? If so, what impact do these differences make on leisure in your life now?

followed by seemingly leading the participant's answer.

Unlike other kinds of interviewing, an ethnographic style of interview develops a life of its own. There is no prescribed order of questions. For example, the description of a typical day sometimes led the conversation towards a discussion about the climate and environment in Canada, compared with that in the participant's home country. A rich description that exceeds the scope of any one question may eliminate the need for a subsequent question. After several interviews and further reading, I added questions about work and home: In what ways do other responsibilities affect whether you are able to do what you like to do? Probing questions often followed: Are you working in your chosen area? Why not? What is it like not to work in your profession? How is the combination of work and home life different in Canada? To identify aspects of life that may affect how 'immigrant women' view and use leisure, I added: What is the most difficult adjustment to make, living here in Canada?

Field notes were used to capture the flavour of the interview, the main issues and to identify questions for future interviews. I drafted a one-page summary of each interview from each set of field notes. Keeping a research journal provided me with a means to critique my interview style and reflect on the relationships I was developing with participants. Occasionally the journal assisted me in working with feelings experienced during the research process. The research journal and notations I made after reviewing many of the transcripts contributed to a process of reflexivity.

Data analysis

The process of data analysis highlights the iterative and inductive nature of interpretation in qualitative research. The data set comprises interview transcripts, field notes written after the interviews, interview summaries and the research journal. The early stages of analysis involved listening to the audiotapes and thinking about the data. Hearing the participants' voices reconfirmed the meaning of the otherwise flat words on the page. Coding the data involved open coding, which reflects the data very closely. This phase of the analysis involved searching for chunks of data that would illuminate the experiences of reconstructing a life in a new country.

I initially worried that the detailed descriptions of daily life that participants recounted were not going to be fruitful in answering the research question. However, the second step of focused coding facilitated recognition of emerging themes and patterns. One of the strongest themes to emerge reflected the complex organization and precise choreography required to manage daily life in a new country. An informal use of initial memos to pursue tentative connections between resettlement and issues raised in the interviews led me back to the literature. Further refinement of the focused coding led to the collapsing of some initial categories of data with others. Four provisional themes are presented here.

FINDINGS

Themes

Orchestrating the day

'It's like we have a parallel computer, doing things, everything is trying to be scheduled in the background, and trying to keep things synchronized … You have to synchronize activities of five people, whereas my husband is just – he can barely keep up his own' (Isabelle). 'Orchestrating' the day (Clark & Jackson 1990, p. 74) brings to mind the image of a conductor with her baton, combining constituent parts to make the whole endeavour succeed. In each description of routines and activities that comprise daily life, it was women who took on this organizational responsibility. In circumstances where both parents worked full-time, women met primary childcare and domestic responsibilities. The disparate countries represented by the women in this sample support gender relations as a way to understand this division of labour, rather than notions of culture alone. That the husbands assisted to varying degrees indicates the fluidity of culture, because it would be unusual for men to cook meals and help with the children in their home countries.

The daily logs that many women completed revealed the number, timing and type of activities that they organized for themselves and their families. Cooking meals, house-cleaning, helping with homework and working outside the home, in paid or volunteer jobs, are familiar activities to Canadian-born mothers with children at home. The feeling of always being in a rush is not unique to women who have resettled in Canada, although it was shared by these research participants. Thus it could be argued that most mothers, especially those working outside the home with primary responsibility for domestic life, have less free time that could be allocated for leisure. The important differences revealed in the data involve the types of activity that comprise the day and how these activities help women to reconstruct a life in Canada.

Activities that lead to improved skills in English took considerable time over the course of a week. Participation in English classes and programmes designed to enhance social integration for immigrants took anywhere from 8 to 15 hours per week. For example, Ling attended English classes four evenings per week and participated in the Building Bridges programme for 3 hours each week, over 12 weeks. This programme offered participants a range of activities to connect them to Canadian society and included an expectation to engage in

volunteer work. Ling volunteers as an English-as-a-second-language (ESL) assistant and plans to complete a course enabling her to teach ESL. Many women talked about watching television to improve their vocabulary. This is a reminder that the type of activity does not necessarily determine its meaning. Watching television meant different things to different women.

From the participants' detailed descriptions of daily life, they apparently have less time for leisure than their husbands. Many participants echoed Fereshteh's sentiment – 'I'm always in a rush!' – and even small changes in daily life contribute to this. Two participants explained that, although they had been middle-income earners in their home country, they had been able to afford domestic help with household chores. In Canada, the combination of earning less and a higher cost of living in a metropolitan area precluded having domestic help. No longer having the support that extended family members once gave also contributes to a busy schedule.

In occupational therapy, the meaning of activities is part of the equation that determines whether the constellation of activities is acceptable to one or not. The responsibility, time and effort required to orchestrate daily life differs for women who come to Canada. This difference is significant for understanding leisure in light of the concurrent themes.

The importance of family

As the first theme implies, family life is currently the core of these women's lives. In trying to understand the meaning of family from the participants' perspectives, I was helped by Maira's discussion about the role of language in constructing identity. This was a particularly interesting comment coming from Maira because she had a background in linguistics and the ability to articulate her thoughts clearly. To explain how functioning in another language changes the way one lives one's life, Maira said: 'You're never yourself because learning another language is not just language. It's mentality and it's everything that goes through language. So you become somebody else when you speak'. It follows that if the social relations of day-to-day life are mediated through language, people are likely to feel most comfortable with family members with whom they also have strong emotional ties. Free time and leisure activities spent with family members far outweighed those done alone or with friends where family members were excluded.

The value placed on family was reflected in how participants spent some of their time. As well, the absence of extended family elicited feelings such as loneliness, depression and being overwhelmed for several women. Extended family relationships were maintained by e-mail, letters, phone calls and, occasionally, visits back home. That visits to Bosnia, Hong Kong and Guatemala were very costly and required considerable savings was offset by the value attached to connecting with family. Ling 'chatted' every Saturday morning with her three brothers in China in 'real time' on the internet. To ensure that her girls knew they were part of a larger family, Rosa and her family visited Guatemala for 6 months. The importance of doing everything possible together as a family was not surprising to hear from Maira and Rosa. Before arriving in Canada as refugees they experienced civil war and had relatives injured and killed. For the other women, the resettlement experience itself and the opportunity to communicate in their first language heightened the importance placed on doing activities with family. As the next theme shows, the significance of family also affected decisions about work.

Work changes

Another way to convey this theme is 'working through the changes'. In one form or other, the women engaged in a variety of work throughout the resettlement process. Only two women were employed in their professions, while the experiences of others included:

- being unemployed due to insufficient English language skills
- working in a job outside their experience and/or education
- doing volunteer work as a step to employment
- working in paid employment primarily out of economic necessity.

Unemployment is not uncommon for immigrants when English is a second language. For three of the four women who were unemployed, proficiency in English was the obstacle. One might speculate that time for leisure would be greater for these individuals. This was not the case. Their days were filled with English classes, seeking out courses to upgrade their skills, and carrying out the gendered family responsibilities described in the first theme.

Most women desired and needed work. However, without Canadian work experience it is often difficult to obtain employment. For this reason, and to further social integration, the women in the resettlement programmes had volunteer jobs. For some – like Ling, who was an ESL assistant – the volunteer job was directly linked to a planned future career. For others, like Fereshteh, volunteer work at the local women's centre and outreach to Iranian women was the closest activity to her profession of social work. There are many benefits to engaging in these kinds of volunteer jobs. Although one woman spoke of enjoying her position, all of the research participants referred to the responsibilities as work. Paid or unpaid work, and work-seeking activities, are time consuming for women who immigrate to this country in ways that differ from the experiences of Canadian-born women. Combined with the importance given to family and orchestrating their activities, there is little time left if we believe that leisure requires free time. The final theme offers the strongest challenge to leisure as an entity divisible from everyday life.

Leisure as socializing

'I think for us, to socialize and share with our friends is our leisure' (Graciela).

The thread of socializing that runs through descriptions of leisure and free time supports the concept of leisure as a dimension rather than a domain of life. Of course, many descriptions of solitary leisure activities were also identified, such as reading in English and their first language. Socializing, however, offered the most consistent means through which intense feelings of pleasure, relaxation and enjoyment occurred. Even women whose English skills allowed a more in-depth discussion of leisure found the idea of leisure as something separate to be inconsistent with their experiences. Rosa explained:

'I guess that the concept of leisure it's not very – you see we don't give a name for things that we do. We just do them. We don't say, "Oh, we're going to have some leisure, or we're going to have a little bit of recreation". We just do things and we never call them by a name, which is very much the northern kind of way – American and Canadian kind of way of giving a name to everything that we do here. We don't in Guatemala … so the concept of leisure is not very clear to me – whether it involves recreation for physical purposes or things like that. So most of the things that we do we call it free time – having our free time together.'

Rosa's comments suggest that leisure does not have identifiable qualities that are not found in other activities or spaces of time. This raises the question of why leisure warrants separate study, yet there has been an increase in academic departments devoted to leisure studies and consequent bodies of literature. For what reason (beyond tradition) does occupational therapy carve leisure out of the daily flow of occupations?

Isabelle's definition gives some currency to a cultural explanation for linking leisure with social activities: 'In the Philippines our leisure activities tend to be more socialized … the activity is the excuse for getting together'. This sentiment was echoed by many of the participants. Isabelle explained the social perspective of leisure as the opposite of what she observed to be the Canadian approach to leisure, where the activity is the central focus. The focus of occupational therapy on leisure as activity is challenged by this evidence – by the participants' experiences. This insight provides preliminary support for conceptualizing leisure as a dimension of social life, not as an occupational performance area.

Cultural differences contribute to this theme, especially for women from countries whose society they define as more group oriented and less individualistic than Canadian society. Cultural differences in the meaning of leisure are evidence that leisure is not a universally understood concept. The role of language contributes particularly to understanding leisure as socializing. The lack of spontaneity that the participants identify in Canadian leisure may prompt women like Graciela and Rosa to start thinking of leisure as something separate. Although social life is shaped by culture, it is an insufficient explanation for the different experiences of this diverse immigrant group. Attributing difference to culture alone erroneously positions culture as something static, rather than a meeting of two cultures and a creation of something new. Socializing may have a different meaning since resettlement, with so much of the interaction one might identify as leisure taking place within the family unit. Time spent in activities such as taking language lessons, accessing resources and looking for work may change the importance of leisure in one's life. This is related to the circumstances of resettlement, not necessarily culture. A discussion of how these themes contribute to theorizing leisure within occupational therapy follows. Not surprisingly for an exploratory study, and in light of the state of knowledge development, more questions are identified than answered.

IMPLICATIONS OF THE FINDINGS FOR THEORY DEVELOPMENT

The problem that prompted this research is occupational therapy's limited, atheoretical understanding of leisure. The study aimed to identify the circumstances of resettlement that contribute to different understandings of leisure held by Canadian-born occupational therapists and women who have immigrated to Canada. The findings intentionally avoid any generalization about 'immigrant women' to avoid reproducing that discourse. Instead, this examination of the daily lives of participants offers evidence of how poorly occupational therapy is served by the current definition of leisure. The definition 'enjoying life' is supported by the findings; this is heartening. Enjoyment or pleasure is a precondition for all activities the women identified as leisure. That knowledge alone, however, does little to define leisure unambiguously and explain its complexity. The role of socializing as a vehicle for leisure was pronounced for the participants. This does not explain leisure but adds a layer of complexity, supported by empirical data. The themes introduced earlier identify three issues that have implications for theory development and practice. To appreciate the potential clinical relevance, picture an occupational therapist interviewing a woman who has immigrated to Canada and who speaks English as an additional language.

First, the therapist will hear the client describe activities strikingly different from those of Canadian-born women. Women who immigrate from non-English-speaking countries take ESL classes, do volunteer work to enhance cultural integration, and attend resettlement programmes – examples of their 'work changes'.

Second, the client and the therapist may attribute different meanings to their activities. Three examples were notable in the data: watching television, reading and taking classes. Watching television is normally 'leisure' if the viewer easily understands the programme. Conversely, watching television in another language may be hard work in the service of learning English and understanding another culture. Responding to the question of what she does for leisure, Ling explained: 'Watching TV means I have to understand what they are talking about, pay attention. So it's a mixed feeling. I quite enjoy watching TV but the other way I feel, I *have* to do it'. Reading has multiple meanings for many of the same reasons.

Taking classes may be seen as leisure for many adults, taken to fulfil an interest or pursue a hobby or upgrade one's education. When immigrants take ESL classes, these are often described as work. Whether these ESL classes fit occupational therapy's understanding of 'work' or function as a survival strategy raises questions about the evidence that supports our notion of 'work'. Proficiency in English increases the likelihood of obtaining paid employment – an objective of all the study participants.

Third, the therapist will hear a wide variance of leisure time available among women who have immigrated to Canada. This variation is influenced by domestic responsibilities, income level and work status. If one cannot work because qualifications or experience are not judged equivalent to Canadian standards, time may be spent upgrading through courses or doing pro bono work to gain Canadian experience. Leaving an environment with inexpensive domestic help and extended family assistance, some immigrants find their time in Canada filled with new responsibilities at home.

Finally, having accurately characterized the client's present mix of activities, the therapist needs to understand how resettlement has affected this mix. A significant change in a client's mix of activities is likely to affect her occupational performance and satisfaction with life.

CONCLUDING THOUGHTS

In conclusion, the findings of this study should prompt occupational therapists to question the evidence on which our understanding of leisure is based. The value placed on family and the responsibility for orchestrating family life described by participants offers evidence that leisure is a dimension of life inseparable from the social relations of everyday life. This challenges the assumption of leisure as an occupational performance area. The research findings show that the participants' activities may be perceived as leisure, when in fact they have different meanings that are shaped by how gender, race and class relations unfold in the context of resettlement. The findings confirm occupational therapy's belief that enjoyment coexists with leisure, but the need for further research to map out the terrain of leisure is clear. The preliminary findings support Reid's (1995) definition of leisure: 'those activities that produce intrinsic rewards and provide the participant with life-enhancing meaning and a sense of pleasure … Leisure, then, is as much of an attitude as it is a type of activity' (p. 14).

ACKNOWLEDGEMENTS

It was my privilege to learn more about leisure through listening to the lives of the 13 women who generously offered their assistance as research participants. The Canadian Occupational Therapy Foundation provided partial funding for this research.

REFERENCES

Badets J, Howatson-Leo L 1999 Recent immigrants in the work force. Canadian Social Trends Catalogue No. 11-008. Statistics Canada, Ottawa

Canadian Association of Occupational Therapists 1997 Enabling occupation: an occupational therapy perspective. CAOT Publications ACE, Ottawa

Clark FA, Jackson J 1990 The application of the occupational science negative heuristic in the treatment of persons with human immunodeficiency infection. Occupational Therapy in Health Care 6(4):69–91

Creese G, Dyck I, McLaren A 1999 Reconstituting the family: negotiating immigration and settlement. Working Paper Series No. 99-10 Research on Immigration and Integration in the Metropolis. Online. Available: http://riim.metropolis.net/ 5 March 2003

Frank G 1992 Opening feminist histories of occupational therapy. American Journal of Occupational Therapy 46:989–999

Katz N 1988 Interest checklist: a factor analytical study. Occupational Therapy in Mental Health 8(1):45–53

Kielhofner G (ed) 1995 A model of human occupation: theory and application. 2nd edn. Williams & Wilkins, Baltimore

Kincheloe JL, McLaren PL 1994 Rethinking critical theory and qualitative research. In: Denzin NK, Lincoln YS (eds) Handbook of qualitative research. Sage, Thousand Oaks, CA; pp. 138–157

Knox S 1998 Evaluation of play and leisure. In: Neistadt ME, Crepeau EB (eds) Willard and Spackman's occupational therapy. 9th edn. Lippincott, Philadelphia; pp. 215–222

Lather P 1991 Getting smart: feminist research and pedagogy with/in the postmodern. Routledge, New York

Ng R 1998 Work restructuring and recolonizing third world women: an example from the garment industry in Toronto. Canadian Woman Studies 18:21–25

Primeau LA 1996 Work and leisure: transcending the dichotomy. American Journal of Occupational Therapy 50:569–577

Reed KL, Sanderson SN 1999 Concepts of occupational therapy. 4th edn. Lippincott, Philadelphia

Reid DG 1995 Work and leisure in the 21st century. Wall & Emerson, Toronto

Rose D, Carrasco P, Charboneau J 1998 The role of 'weak ties' in the settlement experiences of immigrant women with young children: the case of Central Americans in Montreal. Working Paper Series. Joint Centre of Excellence for Research on Immigration and Settlement – Toronto (CERIS). Online. Available: http://ceris.metropolis.net/ 5 March 2003

Said EW 1978 Orientalism. Pantheon, New York

Thobani S 2000 Closing the nation's doors to immigrant women: the restructuring of Canadian immigration policy. Atlantis 24(2):16–26

FURTHER READING

Hemingway JL 1999 Critique and emancipation: toward a critical theory of leisure. In: Jackson EL, Burton TL (eds) Leisure studies: prospects for the twenty-first century. Venture, State College, PA; pp. 487–506

Hiebert D 1998 Immigrant experiences in greater Vancouver: focus group narratives. Working Paper Series No. 99-15 Research on Immigration and Integration in the Metropolis (RIIM). Online. Available: http://riim.metropolis.net/ 5 March 2003

4

Building knowledge through participatory research

Mary Law

OVERVIEW

This chapter outlines the philosophy of participatory research, highlighting the congruence between the fundamental principles underlying both participatory research and client-centred modes of practice. Mary Law describes research undertaken primarily to identify factors that affect the daily activity patterns of children with physical impairments. She demonstrates how a participatory approach to qualitative research assured the relevance of the study, facilitated the translation of findings into action and empowered parents to undertake their own research. Mary shows how the evidence derived from qualitative research can be used both to test and to develop theory, and also illustrates how qualitative evidence can inform policy, research and practice (dimensions that will be addressed further in subsequent chapters).

K.H.

INTRODUCTION

The development of knowledge in any field or discipline is a remarkably non-linear and unpredictable process. Knowledge to inform theory, practice and research emerges from the interactions of ideas within a discipline as they are merged with information from other areas. Dunn & Foreman (2002) have noted that evidence helps to advance knowledge by providing information for immediate use and for informing future research. As they state: 'knowledge development within a professional community requires its members to constantly push the limits imposed by current working paradigms' (Dunn & Foreman 2002, p. 20).

Participatory, qualitative research is particularly suited for the development of knowledge to inform theory, practice and further research in the rehabilitation field. The central focus of the research is to search for an understanding of a specific issue. In this chapter, a particular research example is used to illustrate the generation of evidence in the field of occupational therapy through participatory research. The focus of this research centred on a study of disabling environments that affect the daily occupations of children with disabilities.

PARTICIPATORY RESEARCH

Participatory research is 'an integrated activity that combines social investigation, educational work, and action' (Hall 1981, p. 7). Researchers and citizens work together to examine and solve issues (Kemmis & McTaggart 2000, Park et al 1993). Its predominant characteristics include the active involvement of and control by citizens, empowerment of citizens, a commitment to action and an obligation of the researchers to learn along with the participants.

Participatory research has been practised widely in developing countries as a method to raise the consciousness and improve the living conditions of oppressed citizens (Brown 1986). Researchers and participants work together to define problems, explore alternative solutions and facilitate change. Participatory research is very action oriented, seeking always to empower the participants to make changes to improve their future. It is inherently political, often opposing the status quo, seeking changes in power and economic distribution. Key features of participatory research include research as a social process involving active collaboration of participants, a practical focus, a reflective nature, and a focus on changing both theory and practice (Kemmis & McTaggart 2000).

In participatory research related to disability, the political nature of disability issues and the importance of citizen participation to influence change in our society are recognized (Law & Dunn 1993). In this movement for change, people's personal experiences are united with political action (Oliver & Zarb 1989). Participatory research requires significant changes in power distribution. A suitable definition of power in this context has been proposed by Ferguson (1984), who defines power as 'the ability to act with others to do things that could not be done by individuals alone' (p. 206).

Participatory research is not solely concerned with finding solutions. Rather, it also places importance on the critical analysis of policies and discourse related to the problem and solution (Boggs 1986). Participatory research can be used to elicit and act on people's visions and values. The approach is value explicit, not just descriptive or explanatory. People's ideas and experiences are considered, as well as objective, technical knowledge. In participatory research, the context of a problem and the situations in which it occurs receive great consideration. Issues of disability, for example, are seen as collective problems, caused by the inadequacies of the environments in which we live.

The foundations of participatory research, in contrast to a positivist approach to research, include the acknowledgement that there is no single 'truth', the need for interaction between researcher and participant, and recognition of the importance of the context in which an issue or problem is studied (Kemmis & McTaggart

2000). The participants are actively involved in defining research issues, designing data-collection processes, reviewing analysed data (text) and facilitating change based on the data. While participatory and naturalistic research share many concepts, the key difference between them is the political, action-oriented nature of participatory research. Action towards change is implicit within the participatory research process.

Qualitative, participatory methods can help us to understand complex issues in terms of people's experiences, frustrations and satisfactions (Denzin & Lincoln 2000). This methodology is particularly effective when exploring those complex issues where interrelationships are unclear. In many planning issues, very little is known about what policy and practice issues need to be addressed to improve a complex situation. Participatory research involves citizens directly in an issue, gives them control with available facilitation and empowers them with the skills to work to improve conditions in their community. The process is be driven by their concerns and values.

FIT WITH CLIENT-CENTRED OCCUPATIONAL THERAPY

Occupational therapists, along with many rehabilitation practitioners, espouse the need to engage in client-centred practice. Client-centred practice has been defined as 'an approach to services which embraces a philosophy of respect for, and partnership with, people receiving services' (Law et al 1995, p. 253). Important concepts shared by several frameworks of client-centred practice developed by occupational therapy are outlined in Box 4.1.

An examination of these concepts indicates a striking congruence between the fundamental principles underlying both client-centred practice and participatory research. At the heart of each of these approaches lies a universal respect for persons and the choices that they make on a daily basis. Client-centred practice and participatory research are not techniques but rather are philosophical approaches used to guide practices. The focus of each approach is flexible and

---

Box 4.1 Concepts of client-centred practice

- Respect for clients and their families, and the choices they make.
- Clients and families have the ultimate responsibility for decisions about daily occupations and occupational therapy services.
- Provision of information, physical comfort and emotional support. Emphasis on person-centred communication.
- Facilitation of client participation in all aspects of occupational therapy service.
- Flexible, individualized occupational therapy service delivery.
- Enabling clients to solve occupational performance issues.
- Focus on the person–environment–occupation relationship.

(From Law 1998, with permission of Slack Inc.)

---

centred on the development of a positive collaborative partnership between researchers/service providers and persons experiencing the issues that are the focus of research or service. The provision of information and enablement of persons to solve the issues of concern to them is central to both client-centred practice and participatory research.

One final characteristic that is shared between the client-centred approach and participatory research is the challenge of implementing these concepts on a day-to-day basis. Even if people believe in the principles of these approaches, carrying out these principles is not easy to do. Because of the complex nature of health and human services, implementing services or conducting research in such a way that true partnership is ensured presents a challenge to both persons with disabilities and therapists.

ILLUSTRATIVE RESEARCH EXAMPLE: CHANGING DISABLING ENVIRONMENTS

Childhood physical disability refers to long-term restrictions in the ability to perform daily activities, as a result of a physical impairment such as cerebral palsy, spina bifida or muscular dystrophy. Children with impairments frequently have little control over their day-to-day activities. Their activity patterns differ from those of children without an impairment and reflect more time spent in self-care and passive activities within their home environment than in activities in the community (Brown & Gordon 1987). There are significant environmental barriers in communities that prevent the development of satisfying activity patterns. Environmental constraints include those physical, social, institutional, economic and cultural factors in a child's home, neighbourhood or community that influence participation.

In this research, a broad range of environmental factors that affect the daily activity patterns, participation and integration of children with physical disabilities were studied conjointly. My key interest was the application of planning methods to the management of the environment around children with disabilities and their families. I knew that the experience of parents would be the most valuable source of information about supports and barriers for participation. The study examined the process of bringing together participants, who shared common concerns but did not know one another, in a participatory research project. To that end, the process of the study and the community involvement of the participants during the project were as important as the research outcomes.

The *primary goal* in this research was to identify factors within the environment, family and/or child that affect the daily activity patterns of children with physical disabilities. Together, with parents, I wanted to discover the environmental situations that presented the most substantial challenges to their children. Focus groups and individual interviews were used to gain an understanding of the experiences and difficulties of parents who have a child with a disability. A *second goal* was to examine the use of participatory research in a community and disability context. The parents who participated in this research were the principal architects of the interview probes and the study action process. A *final aim* of the research was to explore and make recommendations with parents about planning strategies that could be used to alter activity patterns and enhance participation.

PARTICIPATORY RESEARCH PROCESS

The study process included four stages: problem identification, data collection, data coding and analysis, and development of theoretical concepts. However, in reality – and as in most qualitative research – the participatory research process used in this study was a cyclical, iterative process, incorporating the establishment of focus groups and the exploration of issues that affect activity patterns, determining how to study these, collecting data, discussing these data, determining actions based on the groups' perceptions and the data, performing actions and evaluating results.

Parents were initially invited to attend one of a series of four focus groups. The purpose of the focus groups was to encourage participants to discuss and identify significant factors that supported or hindered the daily activities of their children. These issues were then used as the basis for individual interviews with all 23 families. Twelve participants agreed to be part of a focus group. The discussion in the groups centred on the 'sorts of things' that made it easier or harder for their children to participate in everyday activities. Issues that were influential in a variety of environmental settings, including the home, neighbourhood, school or nursery, and community, were discussed. Cultural, economic, institutional, physical and social environmental factors were considered. All focus groups and subsequent interviews were audiotaped and later transcribed for analysis. Summaries with textual examples were sent to all focus group participants. Participants were asked to check these for accuracy and were also asked what they wanted to do with the information gathered during the study.

ENABLING PARTICIPATORY RESEARCH TO HAPPEN

Twenty-three families that had a child with an impairment who attended a local children's rehabilitation centre participated in the research. A letter was sent to potential participants from the children's centre and those interested in being a part of the study responded. Once parents had agreed to be part of the study, their names were

---

Box 4.2 Criteria for participation

- Participants controlling agenda
- Participants facilitating change
- Participants helping one another
- Participants continuing to be involved
- Researcher enabling participants to learn new skills

---

given to the researcher. The participants in the study did not know one another at the beginning of the research, nor were they part of any organized group concerned with issues of disability. Because participatory research typically begins with a researcher working with an already existing group, this presented a unique challenge. A number of methods were used to ensure that the entire research process was as participatory as possible and that the parents controlled the directions of the research. These methods included the manner in which the study was introduced and how participants were involved and empowered during the research process.

The principal method used to empower participants to take control of the research process was by means of 'intentional nudging' (see below). The research team had defined criteria by which participation in the research process could be evaluated (Box 4.2). I perceived my role in the research process to be that of a facilitator. This role was described clearly to the participants. I was there to listen to the participants, learn from them, understand their suggestions for change, and help them put ideas into action. Throughout the research process, I tried to ensure that participants were relaxed and comfortable. I listened actively to what they said, often asking questions to probe further into their experiences and ideas. I followed their lead in determining the direction of the interviews. When issues about barriers were raised, I asked for suggestions to change that situation. As well, I often told participants about suggestions already made by other parents.

Maintaining the integrity of the research process

The method used in this research was participatory research, although the participants neither knew one another nor initiated the research project. Despite this limitation, however, the study did meet the criteria that we set for participatory research (Box 4.2). There was active involvement and control by participants, empowerment of participants, a commitment to action and the researchers learned with participants. In terms of the methodology of participatory research, there is evidence from this study that participatory research can work without a preformed citizen group. To work, however, it needed to be executed differently from other participatory research.

The major difference in the process of participatory research with an unformed group was the use of 'intentional nudging' to involve the participants from the beginning and to encourage participant control. Intentional nudging was used during all phases of the study. Features that contributed to the study's participatory nature included the manner in which the research was introduced, how participants were involved from the beginning and how participants were empowered to make decisions about the direction of the research. The research was described to participants as a flexible process: a process where we, as researchers, wanted to explore issues and make recommendations together with participants. I shared experiences with the participants about other research, illustrating how this project would be different. Participants were involved in all aspects of the research and received summaries of focus groups and texts of their interviews. They were encouraged to express their opinions about what should happen at each stage of the project. By the summary meeting, participants felt sufficiently involved to decide to go further. Over the next few months, as their parent group began, they assumed ownership of the process.

RESEARCH FINDINGS

The findings of this study represent the experiences of the participant families, their perceptions of environmental barriers and supports, and their shared experiences in coming together to act on these identified barriers. The findings reflect common themes emerging from the analysis of the stories of these families. The families had many thoughts about their experiences in living with a child with a disability. Their stories form the background against which their perception of environmental barriers and supports and policy solutions can be considered. The themes of 'shattered dreams', 'personal growth' and 'doing it alone' emerged as the most powerful shared experiences of these families.

Parents described initially finding out about a child's impairment as very difficult, but most felt that they had dealt with these difficulties well. In fact, a number of participants eloquently described how having a child with an impairment has caused them seriously to question societal values and had been a positive growth experience for them. While most parents in the study did not express any desire to change their child or their situation, they did clearly state that they must deal with a lot of disability issues on their own.

Primary findings from this research centred on the role that the environment plays in supporting and hindering the participation of children with disabilities in everyday activities. Participants felt that their lives were juxtaposed between two worlds: a world of 'normality' and a world of 'disability'. Parents expressed the concern that the world and community in which they live thinks in terms of normality and perfection when considering children. All parents who participated in the focus groups and/or interviews believed that social attitudes are the biggest handicap for their children. Families stated that they wanted to be viewed as parents first and not only as the parents of a child with a disability. They also want their child to be seen as a child first, not as a 'disabled' child. Participants gained social support primarily through their immediate and extended families.

Many significant physical environmental barriers were identified by the study participants. These barriers ranged from older buildings with stairs and no ramps to new structures such as an accessible creative playground that had a step only 3 metres from the beginning of the creative structure. Participants felt strongly that it was often attitudinal problems or lack of knowledge that prevented physical barriers from being changed or not constructed in the first place.

Institutional environmental factors included barriers and supports associated with the organizations and their representatives or staff that the participants interacted with on behalf of their child. These organizations were diverse and included healthcare facilities, daycare programmes, preschool programmes, schools and school boards, city recreational programmes, sports associations and voluntary, charitable organizations. Parents expressed many frustrations about the time required for them to wade through bureaucracy on behalf of their child. Finding information about programmes was often very difficult. When faced with institutional barriers, participants often found that they had little power to change situations for their children. In many instances, it appeared that the needs of the organization or their staff were placed before the needs of the family and the child with a disability. There were also many instances cited by participants where they had received excellent institutional support. Health workers, school personnel and others had actively asked parents what their choices for their child were and then worked together with them to ensure that the chosen actions were taken. Parents readily identified these kind of people and situations as most comfortable for them. When their opinions were sought and acted upon, parents felt that they had power to influence the process. It was clear that most participants want to act in partnership with organizations and their employees to change conditions for their children.

Specific recommendations for action were developed by participants in this research and subsequently taken to organizations and government as part of discussions to facilitate environmental change. Examples of these policy recommendations given in Box 4.3.

USING RESEARCH EVIDENCE TO INFORM POLICY, THEORY, RESEARCH AND PRACTICE

Informing policy and planning at a local level

It became clear through the research process that most participants wanted to get back together to

Box 4.3 Policy recommendations

Policy suggestions for the community
- Provide educational material and information to City Council and City Administration.
- Increase the visibility and use of accessibility signs in public and private buildings within the community.
- Act to include children with disabilities in community events and in the media.
- Include parents who have children with disabilities in planning activities or other activities that will have an impact on their children's participation in the daily life of the community.
- Encourage parents of children with disabilities to work together to gather resource material about how to deal with their own children's questions and the questions of others about disability.
- Encourage parents to work together so that they may gain greater skills in advocacy and help to change community attitudes.

Policy suggestions for schools
- School Boards should provide information to parents about the process of school placement and parents' rights in that process.
- School Boards should provide support to help parents to choose the appropriate school placement for their child.
- School Boards should review the Identification Placement and Review Committee process to ensure that parents do not feel overwhelmed by these committee meetings and to ensure that parents are full participants.

- School Boards should offer extra resource help and adaptations for children with disabilities as a policy to enable integration.
- Parents and staff at schools should be encouraged to discuss disability issues within their Parent – Teacher Association and parent and staff meetings.
- Issues related to disability should be included in health and lifestyle courses, both in senior public school (ages 12–13) and in high school (ages 14–18).
- School Boards should, on a regular basis, use programmes such as buddy systems and peer helpers to assist children with disabilities in integrating into schools.

Policy suggestions for recreation and other activities done outside the school or home
- The City Activities Guide should be changed to increase the information available to parents about which programmes are available to children with disabilities.
- City recreational programmes, as well as other recreational groups and programmes, should provide a range of options and adaptations so that all children within the community, both those with and those without a disability, can participate.
- Increased training should be available to recreational leaders and coaches about children with a disability and how programmes can be integrated.
- The competitive nature of sports and recreation should be de-emphasized. Children's sports and recreation should emphasize participation and fun for everyone.

share the results of the groups and interviews. A complete summary of this information was sent to all participants along with an invitation to attend a meeting to discuss the results. The summary was organized as a workbook with information about concerns, strategies and suggestions for the future for the most important issues identified by the participants. A blank working section entitled 'Your Ideas for Action' was also included.

A meeting of the participants was held to discuss the study findings. The researcher's role at the meeting was to help participants discuss their ideas and facilitate any actions that were suggested. At the meeting parents decided to form a parent support and advocacy group, prioritize identified issues and work together to change those barriers.

The goals for the group, as formulated at that meeting, included advocacy, information gathering and sharing, and parent training. The group was for all parents of children or adolescents with special needs. Over the next few years, the group met monthly and added new members. The group advocated successfully for the development of improved recreation programmes and has been actively involved in a policy review of programme accessibility for persons with disabilities in the community.

Informing theory

Participatory research can be utilized to test and develop theory. This study, focused on disabling environments, provides an example of both purposes. First, let's examine how a theory was tested through this research.

Over the past two decades, disability advocates have claimed that disability is largely created by the environments in which people who have an impairment live (Jongbloed & Crichton 1990). If our environments foster dependency and poor solutions, then solutions would exist predominantly in planning and social policies aimed at the modification of the environment. The fundamental principle of this approach is the recognition of the ecological nature of disability, and that the problems are caused by the interactions of a child with the environment, not by the impairment itself. Disability is seen as a collective problem, a problem caused by the inadequacies of the environments in which we live (Funk 1987). Social policy would be used as the primary means to increase participation among children with impairments.

This point of view represents a challenge to see disability in a new way. If environments foster dependency, then solutions will exist predominantly in interventions aimed at modification of the environment. However, the substantial effect that environments have on the activities of a child with an impairment is not well understood. Knowledge about the interactions between disability and the environment for children is scant. Disability, activity and environmental factors have rarely been examined together in the past. Rather, the practice has been to examine these factors independently, and to focus predominantly on changing the child, not the environment.

The findings of this study support the proposition that the disability arises from the interaction of the person with an impairment with the environment, and that the predominant barriers to participation that are most easily changed are centred in the external environment. The research findings also provide information about the most important perceived environmental barriers – those that are social, attitudinal and institutional in nature. Having this information enables consumers and practitioners to challenge the common assumption that changing physical environmental barriers is the most important action to improve accessibility. In contrast, the findings from this study indicate that improving accessibility to enhance participation is much more complex than simply eliminating physical barriers.

Let's now look at how the findings from this study have been used to inform and develop theory. As the results of this study began to emerge, I engaged in discussions with colleagues at McMaster University who shared my interests in occupational therapy and environmental issues. We began to meet on a monthly basis, and together explored literature and theories in the fields of occupational therapy, psychology and environment–behaviour studies. Environment–behaviour research includes the disciplines of environmental psychology, sociology, anthropology, human geography and architecture. We were interested in exploring concepts underlying the relationship between persons doing everyday occupations in a variety of environments. Our work led to the development of the Person–Environment–Occupation (PEO) model of practice for occupational therapy (Law et al 1996). This model draws from occupational therapy literature and other multidisciplinary approaches to person–environment relations to describe how persons, as unique, flexible humans, interact with time, space and environments to participate in everyday occupations. Research conducted over the past 6 years has supported the validity and clinical utility of the PEO model (Cooper & Stewart 1997, Green & Cooper 2000, McKye et al 1998, Peachey-Hill & Law 2000, Stewart 1998, Strong 1998, Strong et al 1999, Westmorland et al 2000). The model has also been used to develop and inform practice, as discussed later in this chapter.

Informing research

The process and the findings of this study informed both further research as well as research methods. Two directions of research were stimulated as a result of this project.

The experience of participating in this research study raised questions for myself and others about the process by which parents' support groups emerge and continue. We were particularly interested in parent-led support groups whose goals were friendship and support, provision of information, and sharing experiences. Together with two parent co-investigators, we developed a research proposal that was funded to examine these issues. The focus of the research was to explore parents' perceptions of the outcomes of belonging to a parent-led support group. Findings from that research indicate that these groups are very effective in helping parents to receive information, increase their skills, gain an increased sense of power, and experience a sense of belonging and connection with others who have a child with a disability (Law et al 2001). In this research, we also identified factors such as committed leadership, intimate connections with local community, and flexibility in meeting ongoing members' needs as most important for the development of effective parent-led groups (King et al 2000).

The findings of the participatory research centred on the role that environmental factors play in determining function and participation in everyday occupations. Contrary to expectations, participants did not identify child-related factors such as diagnosis or functional severity as the most important in determining their child's ability to participate in daily activities. Rather, participants identified environmental situations, particularly social and institutional factors (e.g. social attitudes about disability, institutional policies, choice, information, programme support) as the most significant barriers. Although many physical barriers were identified, the participants' experience was that attitudes or lack of knowledge, not lack of technology, prevented these barriers from being changed. Participants recommended that, if health professionals want to help children participate in the activities of childhood, they need to learn more about, and place more focus on, changing environmental factors that support participation.

With the goal to learn more about factors supporting participation, a research group from *CanChild* Centre for Childhood Disability Research at McMaster University gained funding from the National Institutes of Health in the USA for a larger participation study. The primary objective of this multisite project is to undertake a longitudinal study of children with physical disabilities aged 6–14 years (early childhood to adolescence) to determine the child, family and environmental factors that enhance participation in the formal and informal activities of childhood. Innovative methodologies (structural equation modelling and a cross-sequential design) are being used to evaluate the relative contribution of child, family and environmental factors in determining participation of children with long-term, non-progressive physical conditions associated with physical functional limitations in day-to-day activities – conditions such as cerebral palsy, traumatic brain injury and amputations. With a population-based sample of more than 400 children, we are measuring the quantity and quality of the participation of children in the formal and informal activities of childhood and delineating the relative influences of key child, family and environmental factors on the level of their participation. This study is currently ongoing and findings will be available in 2004. The participatory research study described in this chapter was absolutely instrumental in providing information upon which to base this further research.

Participatory research, such as the example described here, can also influence research methods. In this study, parents became an integral part of the study team. Their presence throughout the research process and their involvement in decision-making has led myself and others within our research group actively to include parents as co-investigators on subsequent research studies. Over the past 10 years, since the participatory research study began, I have been involved in at least five other studies in which parents have been full members of the research team. Our research is more relevant, and results move into practice more quickly, as a result of their involvement. In the past 2 years, parents who have been involved in research are now having success in receiving funding for projects that they are leading.

Informing practice

Translating research information into practice is challenging. Many factors affect attempts to change practice: existing attitudes, beliefs and intentions; the quality of training provided; the environment in which change is expected; and the provision of support and follow-up. To be effective, changes to practice must be targeted towards meeting the concerns and needs of service providers. Information must come from credible sources in a way that is usable by practitioners. With that background, I will briefly discuss ways in which the participatory research study described in this chapter played a small but important role in informing practice.

I have already described the PEO model of practice developed by the occupational therapy environmental research group. The members of this group, over the past 8 years, have interacted with many practitioners and participated in many educational events about the PEO model of practice. We have also written an article describing the practical application of the model (Strong et al 1999). These activities appear to have positively influenced the use of the PEO model in practice. Examples of the ways in which this model has been used in practice are outlined in Box 4.4.

The reasons for such extensive use appear to centre on the practical nature of the PEO model as a systematic way to analyse occupational performance over time. By ensuring that analysis of environmental interactions occurs, the model has increased therapists' awareness of its role in causing disability. The model also considers the complexities of human functioning and experience, while expanding the scope of occupational therapy practice, in particular the use of the

environment as a primary focus for intervention. The PEO model facilitates communication amongst practitioners and with clients, and supports client-centred practice.

CONCLUDING THOUGHTS

In reflecting back on this participatory research study, I have been surprised at the many ways in which the research process and findings have influenced future activities. In the course of the study, people's visions and values became apparent, and these provided an effective basis for suggesting policy changes and beginning to achieve action. Participatory, qualitative methods, as used in this study, were particularly useful in chronicling the experiences of people and their interactions in a community context, as well as facilitating change. The process was also more effective in dealing with the complexities of disabling environments because we were able to examine these concerns in an iterative manner. Evidence derived from the study laid the basis for future research, led to greater involvement of parents in research, and influenced the development of an emerging model of practice for occupational therapy.

Box 4.4 Use of the PEO model in practice

- Development of a home support programme in Baffin Island (in Canada's Arctic)
- Development of rehabilitation programmes in Bosnia
- International clinical fieldwork (India)
- Career planning for occupational therapy students (New Zealand)
- School health services (Ontario)
- Workplace re-entry
- A family-centred functional approach to rehabilitation
- New practice guidelines for occupational therapy in Canada
- Basis for modifications to the blueprint for the Canadian Occupational Therapy Certification Examination

REFERENCES

Boggs C 1986 Social movements and political power. Temple University Press, Philadelphia
Brown LD 1986 Participatory research and community planning. In: Checkoway B (ed) Strategic perspectives on planning practice. Lexington Books, Toronto; pp. 123–137
Brown M, Gordon WA 1987 Impact of impairment on activity patterns of children. Archives of Physical Medicine and Rehabilitation 68:828–832
Cooper B, Stewart D 1997 The effect of a transfer device in the homes of elderly women. Physical and Occupational Therapy in Geriatrics 15:61–77
Denzin NK, Lincoln YL (eds) 2000 Handbook of qualitative research. 2nd edn. Sage, Thousand Oaks, CA
Dunn W, Foreman J 2002 Development of evidence-based knowledge. In: Law M (ed) Evidence-based rehabilitation: a guide to practice. Slack, Thorofare, NJ; pp. 13–30
Ferguson KE 1984 The feminist case against bureaucracy. Temple University Press, Philadelphia
Funk R 1987 Disability rights: from caste to class in the context of civil rights. In: Gartner A, Joe T (eds) Images of the disabled, disabling images. Praeger, New York; pp. 7–30

Green S, Cooper BA 2000 Occupation as a quality of life constituent: a nursing home perspective. British Journal of Occupational Therapy 63:17–24

Hall BL 1981 Participatory research, popular knowledge and power: a personal reflection. Convergence 14(3):6–17

Jongbloed L, Crichton A 1990 Difficulties in shifting from individualistic to socio-political policy regarding disability in Canada. Disability, Handicap & Society 5(1):25–36

Kemmis S, McTaggart R 2000 Participatory action research. In: Denzin NK, Lincoln YL (eds) Handbook of qualitative research. 2nd edn. Sage, Thousand Oaks, CA; pp. 567–606

King G, Stewart D, King S et al 2000 Organizational characteristics and issues affecting the longevity of self-help groups for parents of children with special needs. Qualitative Health Research 10(2):225–241

Law M (ed) 1998 Client-centred occupational therapy. Slack, Thorofare, NJ

Law M, Dunn W 1993 Perspectives on understanding and changing the environments of children with disabilities. Physical and Occupational Therapy in Pediatrics 13(3):1–17

Law M, Baptiste S, Mills J 1995 Client-centred practice: what does it mean and does it make a difference? Canadian Journal of Occupational Therapy 62:250–257

Law M, Cooper B, Strong S et al 1996 The person–environment–occupation model: a transactive approach to occupational performance. Canadian Journal of Occupational Therapy 63(1):9–23

Law M, King S, Stewart D et al 2001 The effects of parent support groups for parents of children with disabilities. Physical and Occupational Therapy in Pediatrics 21:29–48

McKye A, Shin J, Letts L 1998 Cultural sensitivity of the person–environment–occupation (PEO) model. Abstract summaries, World Federation of Occupational Therapists Congress

Oliver M, Zarb G 1989 The politics of disability: a new approach. Disability, Handicap & Society 4(3):221–239

Park P, Brydon-Miller M, Hall B, Jackson T (eds) 1993 Voices of change: participatory action research in the United States and Canada. Ontario Institute for Studies in Education, Toronto

Peachey-Hill C, Law M 2000 Impact of environmental sensitivity on occupational performance. Canadian Journal of Occupational Therapy 67:304–313

Stewart D 1998 The transition to adulthood for youth with disabilities: a qualitative exploration. Master's thesis, McMaster University, Hamilton, Ontario

Strong S 1998 Meaningful work in supportive environments: Experiences with the recovery process. American Journal of Occupational Therapy 52(1):31–38

Strong S, Rigby P, Stewart D et al 1999 Application of the person–environment–occupation model: a practical tool. Canadian Journal of Occupational Therapy 66:122–133

Westmorland M, Willams R, Strong S 2000 Workplace perspectives: successful work (re)entry for persons with disabilities (research report). McMaster University, School of Rehabilitation Science, Work Function Unit, Hamilton, Ontario

FURTHER READING

Law M, Dunn W 1993 Perspectives on understanding and changing the environments of children with disabilities. Physical and Occupational Therapy in Pediatrics 13(3):1–17

Smith SE, Willms DG, Johnson N 1997 Nurtured by knowledge: learning to do participatory action research. International Development Research Centre, Ottawa, Ontario

5

Using qualitative focus groups to evaluate health programmes and service delivery

Chris Carpenter

KEY POINTS
programme and services evaluation; participatory research; focus group method; issues of researching disability; ethical issues; spinal cord injury and community living

OVERVIEW

Disability theorists have critiqued the inequitable power dynamics demonstrated by traditional approaches to research into disability issues, in which researchers decide what should be studied, define the parameters of inquiry and determine how the study is conducted, analysed, written up and disseminated. This chapter provides a unique illustration of a research project in which a consumer organization of disabled people contracted Chris Carpenter, a university-based physical therapy researcher, to provide research assistance. Using focus groups, the study accessed the perspectives of members of a disability organization regarding the services provided by that organization. Demonstrating the use of qualitative evidence to inform modes of service delivery, this study also exemplifies the development of partnerships between disability organizations and academic researchers.

K.H.

INTRODUCTION

This chapter describes a qualitative research study that utilized focus groups to evaluate the role of an advocacy organization and the programmes it provides for clients living with spinal cord injury in the community. The focus group method is considered a useful technique for exploring beliefs, understandings and priorities related to illness and disability (Bowling 2002). As such, it offers considerable potential in the evaluation of occupational and physical therapy programmes and interventions, in gaining valuable insight into clients' experiences and perceptions of health and illness, and in exploring complex issues such as the impact of health reforms on practice. However, the focus group method of qualitative research has attracted comparatively little attention in the occupational and physical therapy research literature (Hollis et al 2002, Sim & Snell 1996). In this chapter I discuss the research process and demonstrate how qualitative evidence derived from the focus group method can make an important contribution to health programme evaluation and research. In addition, I examine a number of ethical issues arising from the 'realities' of conducting focus group research and my role as a university-based researcher contracted by a consumer-based organization.

ESTABLISHING THE RESEARCH PRIORITIES AND APPROACH

The research study described in this chapter was conceptualized as the first stage of a systematic evaluation of an advocacy organization that seeks to support individuals with spinal cord injury living in the community through the provision of a diversity of programmes. These programmes are offered in a number of core service areas, such as peer support, respiratory outreach programmes, rehabilitation, educational and vocational counselling, community advocacy and public awareness, transportation, recreation and leisure activities, and independent living and home support. The number and scope of these programmes have expanded over the past decade but little attention has been paid to assessing their effectiveness, and the organization recognized that future programme decisions needed to be more firmly grounded in the current best evidence available.

Health and social services research is concerned with the relationship between the provision, effectiveness and efficient use of health services and programmes, and the health needs or goals of the population. The service users' perspective is a central element in this relationship and, increasingly, researchers have recognized the importance of consistently involving clients in planning and evaluating services (Bowling 2002, Bury & Mead 1998, Krueger 1994, Pope & Mays 1999, Williamson 2001). In exploring possible research approaches, the organization identified a number of priorities that would guide the project. These priorities were: that an open and unbiased discussion of the current and future role of the organization be facilitated with clients, and that clients be the primary source of information.

The organization consulted with different researchers, including myself, in developing an overall research plan. A qualitative methodology was chosen as the most appropriate to reflect the client-centred philosophy of the organization and to address the areas of interest established for this first phase of the evaluative process. These areas of interest are outlined in the next section of this chapter. As a result of my experience as a qualitative researcher and physical therapist specializing in spinal cord injury rehabilitation, I was contracted to conduct the research. I was interested in this project for a number of different reasons – in particular the opportunity to be involved in participatory research in partnership with an organization committed to representing the interests of disabled people.

Disability theorists have vociferously criticized traditional disability research as being structured in relation to the medical or 'individual' model of disability, in which disability is seen as intrinsically related to the person's impairment (Oliver 1993, Stone & Priestley 1996). Research approaches that adopt an objective or neutral stance and are based on the individual model of disability leave disabling personal, practical or political barriers unchallenged and disregard the impact of oppression on disabled people's lives (Moore et al 1998). This criticism applies to qualitative as well as quantitative research (French & Swain 1997). In contrast, adopting the social model of disability as the theoretical underpinning of research leads to the view that disability is socially constructed and that explanations for disablement are to be found within the context of a person's life, rather than within the individuals themselves (e.g. Oliver 1993). Yoshida et al (1998) believe that a shared vision of disability is essential in developing and sustaining effective partnerships between disability organizations and academic researchers. My own understanding of disability had been shaped by the expertise shared with me by individuals who had sustained a spinal cord injury, and I had structured previous research in relation to the social model of disability and the concept of transformational learning (Carpenter 1994). The advocacy organization that spearheaded this project is a proponent of the Independent Living Movement and, as such, it embraces the social model of disability (DeJong 1979). I came to appreciate how important this often taken-for-granted but essential 'shared vision of disability' was to the working partnership we established.

Participatory research is characterized by rigorous evaluation of questions about control: who decides what the research will be about, how it will be conducted, and how thoroughly disabled people are engaged in decision-making about the project and its outcomes (Zarb 1995). Our 'shared vision' made it easier to incorporate these key principles into the research design and process. The involvement of participants at every stage of the research ensures that the process and products remain socially relevant, and facilitates the production of knowledge as socially relevant

information that is usable to both participants and researcher (Yoshida et al 1998). This project was essentially a client-generated one to which I was able to contribute a specific set of skills and abilities. This contribution consisted of recommending the focus group method, coordinating the data collection, analysing the data and generating a report outlining the findings and subsequent recommendations. My responsibility, as I saw it, was to facilitate a rigorous research process in order to ensure that the 'evidence' generated would be trustworthy and transferable and, thereby, of benefit to the organization's clients.

THE CHOICE OF FOCUS GROUPS AS QUALITATIVE METHOD
Advantages of focus groups

Focus groups are frequently defined as 'group interviews' centred on a specific topic (Hollis et al 2002, Sim & Snell 1996). However, this definition could include other categories of group interviews, such as nominal or Delphi groups (see Ch. 11), both of which, according to Morgan (1997), are 'manifestly different from focus groups' (p. 6). What differentiates the focus group approach is the core component in data collection of 'group interaction'. Participants are most frequently brought together on the basis of some shared experience and encouraged to interact with each other rather than the group facilitator and, in this way, create an audience for one another. The participants in this study differed from one another in terms of their age, life experience and socio-economic status, but they all shared the reality of living with spinal cord injury in the community. The use of group dynamics is viewed as one of the advantages of focus groups (Bowling 2002) in stimulating discussion, generating a broad spectrum of ideas and facilitating insights, particularly when the topic is 'either habit-ridden or not thought out in detail' (Morgan 1997, p. 11). According to Barbour & Kitzinger (1999), this method allows participants 'to generate their own concepts and questions, pursue their own priorities on their own terms using their own vocabulary' (p. 5).

The focus group method involves multiple participants and so facilitates the collection of a relatively large amount of data on a topic in a limited period of time. This was considered a particularly useful characteristic for this exploratory research study. However, there is a trade-off related to the decreased depth and detail of information obtained in comparison with one-to-one interviews (Morgan 1997). Researchers face the choice between giving control to the group and possibly learning *less* about the specific topic of interest, or being more directive and perhaps learning *more* while at the same time losing the free-flowing discussion considered to be a defining characteristic of focus groups (Morgan 1997). Group discussions make it easier to adopt a less structured approach and facilitate a more relaxed research atmosphere and, as a result, may be more conducive to obtaining in-depth as well as sensitive information (Barbour & Kitzinger 1999, Bowling 2002).

This 'freer' and more dynamic situation does, however, require considerable skill on the part of the group facilitator (Barbour & Kitzinger 1999). Examples of such skill include the ability to encourage all members of the group to participate, to balance talking and asking questions to stimulate the group interaction with keeping quiet, and to remain engaged with the discussion in order to clarify ambiguous statements and monitor the group dynamics.

Limitations of focus groups

The constitution of the group is frequently an unknown quantity and the group process may give an advantage to those participants for whom sharing 'private' opinions and confronting others' viewpoints may be easier. The heightened visibility of the group facilitator and potential for exerting a constraining influence on group interaction has been cited as a disadvantage of focus groups. However, as Barbour & Kitzinger (1999) point out, these concerns also apply to other qualitative methods such as one-to-one interviews and participant observation, and, in fact, group work may 'dilute' the effect of the facilitator's persona.

Box 5.1 Areas of research interest

- Explore with clients their experiences of living with disability in their communities, specifically in relation to reintegration and participation.
- Identify how individual client goals in the areas of, for example, health, employment, leisure and education are supported or restricted within their community.
- Identify how the organization currently contributes to the achievement of these goals and how it might contribute in the future.

After weighing the advantages and limitations outlined in the literature, we decided that focus groups would be the most useful method of investigating the three areas of interest identified by the organization (Box 5.1).

THE RESEARCH PROCESS

Recruiting and involving the participants

Ten focus groups were conducted in five different geographical locations in British Columbia. Individuals living with spinal cord injury in these communities were invited to participate by local regional consultants employed by the organization and through a flier mailed with the announcement of a forthcoming conference. A number of issues relating to recruitment quickly became apparent once I began to conduct the focus groups. I was primarily dependent on local regional representatives of the organization to contact potential participants. MacDonald & Fudge (2001) recommend that researchers form 'partnerships with any consumer, community or advocacy groups that are affiliated with the desired participants, especially if the topic is sensitive' (p. 120). However, I had some ethical concerns about representatives of the organization who had commissioned the research study being involved in recruiting potential research participants, and I will discuss these concerns in more depth below.

Participation in the focus groups required individuals to travel to a common venue and coordinate with others, such as support personnel, family

Table 5.1	Profile of the participants		
	Women (n = 19)	Men (n = 48)	Total (n = 67)
With disability	11	44	55
Spinal cord injury	8	43	51
Other	3	1	4
Family member, friend or caregiver	8	4	12

members or friends. Any expenses accrued, for example associated with transportation or support personnel, were reimbursed. As lunch or dinner was served before each focus group, many of the participants naturally assumed that those who accompanied them were invited not only to the meal but also to participate in the focus group discussions. I, on the other hand, arrived at the *first* focus group under the impression that only individuals with spinal cord injury would be participating in the discussion. This eventuality had not been addressed in the planning stages. As a result, family and friends also participated in the focus groups. These individuals brought different and equally important perspectives to the discussions (see Table 5.1 for a profile of the focus group participants).

Regional consultants, assuming that some participants might not be able to attend, had sensibly recruited more participants than would be needed. Morgan (1997) recommends over-recruiting by 20% for no-shows; however, he gives no advice to researchers in the event that 'no-shows' are not the problem. On two occasions, nearly double the number of people theoretically required to conduct a focus group attended the venue (see next section for a discussion of group size and composition). As the researcher, excluding some of these individuals from participating in a focus group did not seem to me to be an option. The 'extra' participants had come assuming that they would make a contribution to the study and I felt it was important to acknowledge them and give them the opportunity to participate in the discussion. Fortuitously, on both occasions, a representative of the organization had accompanied me to the venue *and* I had an extra tape recorder with me,

so in these locations I decided to run a second focus group. However, using the organization's representative as a group facilitator raised some ethical issues, given that we were exploring the role of the organization and the focus group participants were potentially, if not actually, recipients of the services offered by the organization.

The literature recommends that the room in which the focus group is held be quiet and comfortable, free from interruptions and protected from observation by those not involved in the research (Barbour & Kitzinger 1999). As the researcher travelling to the venues, I had little or no choice about these details. However, as luck would have it, the arrangements made by the regional consultants – involving community centres, restaurant and hotel meeting rooms, a church hall and a college seminar room – proved appropriately private, 'informal' and comfortable. Increasingly, as the research process unfolded, I recalled the following words of wisdom that qualitative focus group researchers need to be 'flexible' and 'able to think on their feet'; 'avoid presenting themselves as experts'; and be 'sensitive' to the participants' experience (Barbour & Kitzinger 1999, Morgan 1997).

Position of the researcher

I assumed the role of group facilitator in eight of the ten focus groups conducted for this study. As with other qualitative methods, it is important to consider how the researcher is located in relation to the participants and, in this case, the organization being studied. I was not employed or connected with the organization and, with the exception of three individuals, had not met any of the participants before. As a clinician and researcher I had an in-depth knowledge of spinal cord injury and the issues related to living with disability in the community, and had considerable experience moderating groups. This knowledge and experience enabled me to follow the discussion, to understand the 'insider' vocabulary used by the participants and to ask probing questions as required, and it also contributed to the interpretive decisions I made in analysing the data. However, as an able-bodied researcher involved in disability research, I had no expertise in living on a day-to-day basis with a disability and was dependent on the participants to choose the information they considered important for me to know about managing a disability in the community and over many years.

Group size and composition

The group size and composition depends on the purpose of the research and the research reality confronting the researcher (Barbour & Kitzinger 1999, Morgan 1997). In this study I assumed a high level of interest in the topic on the part of the participants and I was interested in ensuring that all the participants would have the opportunity to share their perspectives with the group. Morgan (1997) suggests that, as a 'rule of thumb', group sizes below six may make it difficult to sustain a meaningful discussion and a group of more than 10 may prove difficult to manage (p. 43). In this study the group size varied between six and 12 participants, and a total of 67 people were involved in the study.

Most authors recommend conducting between three and five groups (Barbour & Kitzinger 1999, Bowling 2002, Morgan 1997). This recommendation is based on the claim 'that more groups seldom provide meaningful new insights' (Morgan 1997, p. 43) or, in other words, continued data collection no longer generates new understanding or insights about the research topic. In this study I had planned to conduct eight focus groups and, as described above, we conducted an additional two groups. While it could be claimed that the participants shared the experience of living with a spinal cord injury, I felt it was important to compare how community contexts, not just the larger urban centre, influenced those experiences. In order to capture these different perspectives, I felt that more groups would be required to achieve 'data saturation' (Glaser & Strauss 1967).

Another 'reality' of focus group research is that the 'precise composition of focus groups will often be a product of circumstance rather than planning' (Barbour & Kitzinger 1999, p. 8). In this study 'circumstance' proved advantageous. The groups

formed in this study consisted of a mix of those who knew one another well, those who were merely acquainted and those who were new to everyone. In this way they represented the networks in which people with spinal cord injury normally discuss the type of disability issues raised in this research study – or what Barbour & Kitzinger (1999) call the 'naturally occurring' group. These authors suggest that this type of group is one of the most important contexts in which ideas are formed, information shared and decisions made. Participants frequently commented that they had found the discussions useful and enjoyable in terms of forging new connections, stimulating new options and providing useful information, and suggested that these types of 'get-together' be organized on a regular basis.

A purposive or 'theoretical' sampling approach (Glaser & Strauss 1967) was adopted in this study. This type of sampling aims to encompass diversity and involve people with expertise in the topic being studied, and is guided by the research questions being posed. Given that more men sustain spinal cord injuries, I was concerned in case the perspectives of women with disability would not be represented in the study. I did not, however, act on those concerns by suggesting to the regional consultants that they specifically solicit women participants, and, once again, 'circumstance' proved advantageous (see Table 5.1).

Data analysis and presentation

The focus group discussions were audiotaped and augmented with notes taken during and after each group. The tapes were transcribed using the services of an experienced transcriber. The data analysis involved me listening to the tapes, re-reading the transcripts and 'indexing' sections of each transcript that, in my opinion, appeared to inform the goals of the research. I summarized this content using different words or phrases to represent emerging themes within that focus group discussion. These words or phrases became familiar as they occurred in other focus groups. I also found Morgan's (1997) concept of 'group-to-group validation' (p. 63) useful in guiding my analytical decisions. This concept, according to

Morgan (1997), involves taking into consideration a combination of three factors: 'how many groups mentioned the topic, how many people within each of these groups mentioned the topic, and how much energy and enthusiasm the topic generated among the participants' (p. 63). The findings were presented in the form of a 'final' report in which I attempted to achieve a balance between direct participants' quotations and a descriptive account of the themes.

SUMMARY OF THE RESEARCH FINDINGS

Living in the community

The participants were asked to explore their experiences of reintegration and participation in their communities and the factors that supported or constrained these experiences. The themes that emerged represent topics that were consistently raised within groups and by all the groups. They are not presented here in any particular order of importance, but what is evident is the degree to which they overlap and interconnect.

'Can't afford to go to work'

'I like to work – it's what people in society do, but with a disability if you go to work you're penalized for it.'

The participants described a system made up of a patchwork of public programmes that are not designed to function in a coordinated way. Pension plan and welfare guidelines stipulate that recipients cannot earn any income beyond a minimal exemption without it being completely 'clawed back'. This acts as a barrier for people wishing to work part-time or on a contractual basis. In addition, such employment rarely includes the benefits available through government assistance. Loss of dental, drug and other benefits would be especially costly to disabled people. All the groups discussed the burden of disability-related expenses, including personal assistants, wheelchairs, cushions, medications, medical supplies and vehicles, and viewed these as being poorly understood by the rest of society and particularly by policy-makers. Government policies dictating that financial support not be provided to individuals with disability until all other sources of funding have been exhausted were described as 'demoralizing', 'unfair', and 'discriminating against disabled people'.

'Flexible home support is the key'

'I'm in a share care situation – you live a very regimented life. I can't have someone come at 10.30 p.m. one night and 9.30 p.m. the next, or change my mind on a daily or even weekly basis. I'm stuck with the schedule.'

The ability to manage their own daily lives by employing and directing their own personal care assistants was identified as a critical factor in enabling full participation in community living. Successful self-managed care was seen as providing the opportunity for flexibility in scheduling and self-care routines that adapted to their lifestyles rather than the opposite. The responsibility of hiring, training and keeping care assistants consumed a great deal of time and energy. The difficulties experienced in finding and retaining the right person were seen as drawing attention to the vulnerability inherent in living with a disability. Accessing personal care staff through an agency represented considerably less flexibility and freedom of movement. A recent proposal to downsize and withdraw funds from the Ministry of Health's provision of individualized funding to people with disabilities was a serious cause for concern.

'You've got to feel good about yourself'

'Life is generally good, probably because we choose to make it that way. No different from anyone whether you're in a chair or not – it's up to you to make what you can of it.'

The participants emphasized the importance of taking personal responsibility for their own lives. A sense of well-being was associated with being able to make choices and pursue interests that resulted in a sense of achievement and satisfaction, or just simply 'getting out and doing something every day'. The advocacy organization was seen to contribute to them 'getting on with it' by providing essential information when needed, by being, as one participant said, 'the yellow pages of disability'. Volunteering was an important contributor to a sense of purpose, and the activities described included involvement with community organizations, local government committees, fundraising, amateur sports, theatre groups, and teaching literacy and computer skills. Social isolation was identified as a major contributor to poor quality of life.

The role of family and friends

'It [being injured] really makes you sort out what is important. I'd never have made it without my family and friends.'

Family and friends were described as providing indispensable emotional and practical support in both the rehabilitation stage and over 'the long haul'. Family members, particularly spouses or partners, described the strain of supporting the individual's reintegration into the community combined with the caregiving role, and the changes experienced in their relationship as a result of the injury and subsequent disability. These stresses were exacerbated by a lack of peer or professional support and, in some cases, inadequate home care support and changed financial status. Participants discussed how other things, for example travelling, sexual activity, having children, sustaining a relationship and keeping fit, became important once they had established themselves at home. However, they found it difficult to access information or professional resources that could assist them in addressing these issues.

Networking with peers

'Most of the stuff I taught myself by trial and error. You've got to talk to others, particularly people who have been in chairs a long time. They can tell you so much.'

All the groups discussed the support they gained from others who shared the experience of spinal cord injury, and expressed their willingness to assist others with less experience than them. These important networking activities included assisting newly injured individuals to make the transition from rehabilitation to the community by linking them with 'an old hand' in their local community who could provide moral support and act as a role model for living with disability. All the participants valued networking because of the opportunities it gave them to exchange information, particularly related to purchasing equipment, managing health problems, and accessing appropriate funding or education resources and recreation opportunities in local areas.

Accessing resources and information

'So much time is spent trying to find out stuff about employment, retraining – that sort of thing. It's really hard to get information. All depends on lucking into someone in the know.'

The groups identified a diversity of organizations and agencies whose services were of assistance to them in going back to school, preparing for employment or enhancing mobility. Accessing these useful resources was generally considered to be the result of 'trial and error' – a 'hit and miss' process dependent on 'who you knew' or 'happened to talk with'.

'I'm tired of coming in the back door'

'It's a small community, so I understand the wheelchair users aren't exactly first on the list, but still I get tired of coming through the kitchens and past the garbage.'

The participants agreed that there had been considerable improvement in environmental accessibility over the past 15 years but that the real mobility benefits in terms of curb ramps and paved sidewalks depended on where in the province they lived and the commitment of the municipal governments. The participants were fully aware of the National Building Code that provides minimum standards of safety and design of public and rental buildings. However, they gave numerous example of buildings, including 'the only dental office in the place', that were inaccessible or when 'access' would require them 'to enter through the kitchen' or 'be hauled up the stairs'. There was an overall concern that public building alterations 'have not gone far enough', that they were not enforced with any consistency and that people with disabilities were not being involved in ensuring that access decisions were realistic and appropriate.

Transportation and parking

'The fact that you have to plan so many days in advance, get picked up hours before, kills all spontaneity. It means you can't socialize like a regular person – it kills self-esteem.'

Transportation problems described by the participants related to the scarcity or non-existence of options. In some areas accessible transit was limited, for those who did not own their own vehicle, to subsidized para-transit services, such as the 'Handy-Dart' non-profit scheme. This service provides a useful option, but there are problems associated it. The service has to be booked in advance, rides may be shared between a number of passengers, and priority is given to those keeping medical appointments or going to work. In Vancouver, other transportation options exist that are not available in the rest of the province, such as accessible buses on many routes, the SeaBus and SkyTrain systems, and accessible taxis. These provide welcome choices but concerns were raised about drivers' lack of safety awareness and negative attitudes towards passengers with disabilities. Participants who drove their own vehicles, regardless of which community they lived in, identified parking as a significant problem. The main issue could be encapsulated by the question asked by one of the participants: 'Who *doesn't* have a handicapped sticker?'.

Rehabilitation and medical services

'There are really no resources in my community. Once you leave rehab, you're on your own.'

The information and support given to them and their families at the rehabilitation centre were much appreciated by those participants who had sustained a spinal cord injury in recent years. However, the length of stay in rehabilitation is short and the participants expressed concerns at the lack of follow-up and support once they had been discharged into the community. The participants gave a clear message in their discussions that more education and information in their communities was needed to help them maintain healthy lifestyles and manage medical problems effectively. Participants articulated concerns about the general lack of knowledge about spinal cord injury-related problems on the part of their physicians and other health professionals, and the difficulty in accessing rehabilitation specialists when needed.

Keeping fit and staying healthy

'I can definitely say, without a doubt, that working at the local fitness centre is the one thing that has really changed my life.'

Participants were clearly aware of the desirability of keeping fit and maintaining a healthy lifestyle. They identified a diversity of fitness and recreational activities that they felt contributed to their health, for example wheelchair racing, exploring the provincial parks, swimming, camping and going to the gym. A number of barriers to their involvement in a regular exercise programme were identified, such as the perception that fitness groups and pool administrators were concerned that wheelchair users represented a legal risk. In many communities, fitness facilities were simply not available or owners were unwilling either to make their facilities accessible or to accommodate individual needs.

Computer access and proficiency

'My computer opens up the whole world. You can find out anything. You don't need to ask anyone.'

The participants described themselves as being at various levels of computer literacy, and some had not yet acquired the technology. They all shared the opinion that computers can play an important role in disabled people's lives. Participants who were 'online' accessed information, contacted resources, traded stocks, communicated with friends, designed things with others, conducted their businesses and joined chat rooms. The groups identified that purchasing computer hardware often presented a problem and that it was essential for the beginner to have access to reliable technological support in order to become computer proficient.

RECOMMENDATIONS

The focus group participants were also asked to consider what the advocacy organization 'might look like in the future' and what programmes or services might most effectively support them in their communities. The following recommendations represent a summary of their discussions. It was recommended that the organization:

- allocate more resources and funding to decentralize the organization and support the role of the regional consultant within specific communities
- maintain personal contact between organizational representatives and individuals with disability both during rehabilitation and over the long term in their communities
- facilitate interaction and sharing of information within local communities through purposeful social events, such as education seminars, equipment showcases and fundraising events
- facilitate peer and group support for those – spouses, partners and children – who live with a person with disability
- consult with the regional membership to identify issues and take a stronger, more proactive, advocacy role in both local and provincial arenas
- assume a leadership role in collaborating with other special interest disability groups in lobbying government on disability issues
- devote resources to developing and maintaining a website as a comprehensive and current resource for clients
- collaborate with the rehabilitation centre and other healthcare resources in disseminating health and medical information to family practitioners and in promoting quality of health care throughout the province for individuals with spinal cord injury
- form partnerships with fitness and community centres in developing accessible facilities and encouraging people with

disabilities to participate in exercise and healthy lifestyles.

ETHICAL ISSUES ARISING FROM THE STUDY

Qualitative methods provide researchers with the tools to explore clients' beliefs and value systems and the meanings with which they make sense of their lives and experiences (Hammell & Carpenter 2000). Systematic qualitative research has a potentially significant contribution to make to evidence-based practice (Ritchie 1999) and to client-centred practice and theory (Rebeiro 2000). However, qualitative research approaches are not, by definition, client-centred. To ensure that disability research is non-exploitative and participatory, and that it promotes disabled people's agendas, researchers need to engage in critical reflection on the ethical implications of their research (Moore et al 1998). This section represents my own reflections on the ethical implications of this study.

Focus group work often involves increased dependency on gatekeepers (Barbour & Kitzinger 1999). In this study the regional consultants acted as gatekeepers in that they solicited *and* screened potential participants, and made all the room and catering arrangements. As employees of the organization that commissioned the study, they inevitably influenced the research process. However, in reality, I was unable to find a practical way of circumventing the regional consultants. They recognized the conflict that their presence at the venues represented and were happy to comply with my suggestion that they neither socialize with the participants before the focus groups nor participate in them. The regional consultants received a brief explanation of the purpose of the research study but it became clear that, in reality, different interpretations of this information were being passed on to potential participants. As a result, participants who attended the venues had different understandings of the purpose of the study and why they had been invited. Consequently, it became imperative that I provide some background information about the study, explain the focus group method, and give each participant the opportunity, should they wish, to withdraw. In fact, all the participants chose to be involved. The explanations offered at the beginning of each focus group and a taped verbal agreement from each participant served as informed consent in this study. With hindsight, it would have been preferable if I had contacted the potential participants before arriving at the venue. In this way the information disparities could have been offset and a confidential informed consent obtained.

As Barbour & Kitzinger (1999) point out, focus group participants, unlike interviewees, 'cannot be given an absolute guarantee that confidences shared in the group will be respected' (p. 17). I attempted to address any confidentiality concerns the participants might have by establishing some ground rules prior to the group discussion. I also assured them that only the transcriber and myself would have access to the audiotapes and transcripts, and that their names would not be documented on the transcripts or in the final report.

As a result of my experience interviewing individuals with spinal cord injury in a previous study (Carpenter 1994), I anticipated that during the course of the group discussion participants might provide one another with misinformation. Such information might then be implicitly legitimized by my presence as the researcher. As Barbour & Kitzinger (1999) point out, it would be inappropriate for the researcher, under these circumstances, to leave the group with such misunderstanding. In such instances, I believed it was my responsibility as the researcher to provide timely and accurate information. In reality, the situation did not arise. Considerable exchange of information did occur, but group members were well informed and when necessary provided correction and clarification to one another.

I experienced one conflict resulting from my partnership with the organization that had commissioned the study. This conflict existed between my responsibility as researcher to meet the needs of the organization and my desire to maintain the integrity of the individual participant–researcher relationship. I have come to believe that researching disability issues requires a commitment to certain core principles related to the concepts of reciprocity and representation. Reciprocity 'implies

give and take, a mutual negotiation of meaning and power in the research process' (Carpenter & Hammell 2000, p. 116). In forming a partnership with the disability organization based on mutual agreement and shared values, I had assumed that reciprocity had been addressed. What I had not anticipated was the lack of control I would have in maintaining the integrity (as I perceived it) of my direct relationship with the focus group participants. Ideally I would have preferred to involve the participants throughout the research process in reviewing the emerging themes or providing feedback on the report or their experience of the research process, but because funding was limited these strategies were not deemed practical. I was eager, however, to facilitate follow-up communication and sharing of information between the participants and the organization. To that end, I had proposed sending each of the participants a copy of the final report and I planned to publish a synopsis of the findings in the organization's newsletter with a general acknowledgement of the participants' contributions. During the planning phase I had understood that these plans were acceptable to the organization, but at a later date these strategies were vetoed. The reasoning was that 'they might bias the results of further research initiatives'. A research advisory committee, involving people with and without disabilities, represented the organization in our deliberations on the research project. They clearly understood the role of the organization in representing the interests of disabled people throughout British Columbia, and their decisions were based on a broader research plan and the ultimate benefits of this research to the disabled population. My concern related to the role of the researcher in qualitative research in utilizing strategies such as member-checking to ensure full representation of the participants and the trustworthiness of the research. The conflict I experienced emphasized to me the importance of ensuring a full articulation of expectations and negotiation of a shared agenda early in the research partnership between disability organizations and academic groups or individuals.

The concept of representation 'raises questions of how accountability is established (and to whom we, as researchers, aim to be accountable)' (Carpenter & Hammell 2000, p. 116). Moore et al (1998) outline a number of core rights that they feel disabled people involved in research are entitled to and that embody this concept of representation. These include 'rights of access to the process of research (planning, carrying out, dissemination), entitlement to set agendas, to describe their own experiences and to have personal experience valued. Rights to confidentiality, ownership of data, to ask for account to be taken of one's views in implementation of policy and practical changes arising from the research, and the right to understand the nature of the research and to reject research' (p. 16). As an academic researcher, I had struggled in previous projects to be accountable to research participants in ensuring these rights and to break down the traditional relationships of power between research participants and researchers. The expertise of living with a disability has not been widely acknowledged as important within the 'scientific' community, and qualitative research exploring this expertise has been subsumed by the 'received' quantitative research paradigm which places the emphasis on solving intrinsic, biological or functional problems of individuals living with long-term health issues. This academic perspective on disability as solely a clinical phenomenon negates the full participation of people with disabilities (Yoshida et al 1998). Furthermore, disability researchers within the academic environment are influenced by many factors, such as the interests and policies of funding agencies, professional monitoring and evaluation procedures, career enhancement and personal growth. Some of these factors exert more pressure than others and detract from researchers developing alternative approaches to disability research.

Working in partnership with a disability organization alleviated many of my previous concerns about representation. The organization represents a collective experience of disability issues ranging from personal experiences with rehabilitation to community living issues and political advocacy. The research was initiated as a result of this experience and predicated on the expertise of disabled people living in the community, and the research outcomes were used directly to benefit the participants and others with disabilities and to generate further research.

CONTRIBUTION OF THE FINDINGS TO PROGRAMME PLANNING AND RESEARCH

Health services evaluation is usually based on the collection of data about the structure, process and outcomes of services or programmes (Bowling 2002). Structure refers to the organizational framework for the activities; process refers to how the service is organized, delivered and used; and outcome refers to the impact (effectiveness and appropriateness) of the activities of interest in relation to individuals and communities (Bowling 2002). Few investigators who have employed epidemiological methods have succeeded in taking these variables, and their interplay, into account (Bowling 2002). Indeed, epidemiological methods are not designed to cope with these complexities (Baum 1995). However, the findings of this qualitative study address all three components of service delivery in terms of understanding what is important and relevant in the community context and to the individuals who live with disability in that context, and how the organization's role is perceived by the clients it supports. The evidence generated by this study has been used by the organization to modify specific programmes, such as the recently created peer support programme, and to enhance others, such as the outreach education programme. The participants indicated that the organization needed to market better the existence of the peer support programme in order that clients might both benefit from the service and become involved as peer mentors. These marketing strategies have already resulted in more clients being involved in both capacities.

A strong argument is now being made for the 'stand alone' nature of the evidence generated through rigorous qualitative studies in health care (Baum 1995, Bowling 2002, Pope & Mays 1999, Sofaer 1999). The organization clearly endorsed this argument in acting quickly to implement changes based on the evidence generated from the study. It was also clear that the organization needed to draw on a spectrum of qualitative and quantitative approaches if service policies and delivery were to be based on the 'best' available evidence (Baum 1995, Bowling 2002, Campbell et al 2000, Goering & Streiner 1996, Morgan 1998). As a result, this study was conceived as part of a larger evaluative project and the next phase will employ a quantitative research approach in the form of a cross-sectional descriptive survey.

There is considerable evidence that focus groups can contribute substantially to the creation of surveys (Barbour 1998, Bowling 2002, Goering & Streiner 1996, Morgan 1998). This survey is currently being constructed and the findings of the focus group study are being used to ensure that all the domains that need to be measured in the survey are captured rather than relying on the researcher's assumptions about what is relevant. In addition, the richness of the focus group data is contributing to the generation of items that fully cover the content of each domain and that incorporate the language and vocabulary used by the focus group participants. In this way, the accessibility and relevance of the survey will be enhanced and differences in how the respondents interpret the questions will be minimized (Morgan 1998). Evidence from both the focus group and survey research studies will be used to make recommendations for the implementation of enhanced or new programmes, the outcomes of which can then be rigorously evaluated.

CONCLUDING THOUGHTS

A review of the history of public health and community service delivery highlights the serendipity of both programme development and implementation. Decisions concerning service delivery and programme planning are invariably influenced by the ebb and flow of political agendas and events, by the changing priorities of the community and individuals, and by innovations in health care – and rarely on the basis of evidence derived from rigorous research (Baum 1995). Programme design, implementation and evaluation are considered essential competencies for occupational therapists and physiotherapists (Canadian

Alliance of Physiotherapy Regulators, Canadian Physiotherapy Association & Canadian University Physical Therapy Academic Council 1998, Canadian Association of Occupational Therapists 2002). However, rehabilitation service delivery research is an aspect of evidence-based practice that suffers from a paucity of evidence to direct how and where rehabilitation practice should be delivered (Law 2002). The project described in this chapter illustrates that qualitative research methods have a significant contribution to make, both separately and in combination with quantitative research approaches, to the evaluation of rehabilitation programmes and services. Evidence-based rehabilitation practice must draw its evidence from multiple sources to be of real benefit to clients. However, without input from the people with experience of disability or illness and for whom services are being planned, a real gap remains in our understanding that undermines our ability to deliver client-centred practice. As a researcher, I recognize that the challenge lies in investigating and documenting evidence derived from qualitative research methods in a manner that meets the criteria of rigorous 'good' research (Krefting 1991). Participatory research involves forming collaborative partnerships between researchers, service providers and rehabilitation consumers, individually or in groups, and offers a means of evaluating services or programmes in a way that focuses on the dynamics of the process and is consumer-driven.

ACKNOWLEDGEMENTS

I am grateful to the many people throughout British Columbia who were willing to contribute their expertise and knowledge to this study and to Bert Forman, Director of Rehabilitation Services, for his support.

REFERENCES

Barbour R 1998 Mixing qualitative methods: quality assurance or qualitative quagmire? Qualitative Health Research 8(3):352–361
Barbour R, Kitzinger J 1999 Conducting focus groups. In: Barbour R, Kitzinger J (eds) Developing focus group

research: politics, theory and practice. Sage, London; pp. 2–19

Baum F 1995 Researching public health: behind the qualitative–quantitative methodological debate. Social Science and Medicine 40(4):459–468

Bowling A 2002 Investigating health and health services. 2nd edn. Open University Press, Philadelphia

Bury T, Mead J (eds) 1998 Evidence-based healthcare: a practical guide for therapists. Butterworth Heinemann, Oxford

Campbell S, Roland M, Buetow S 2000 Defining quality of care. Social Science & Medicine 51:1611–1625

Canadian Alliance of Physiotherapy Regulators, Canadian Physiotherapy Association, Canadian University Physical Therapy Academic Council 1998 Competency profile for the entry-level physiotherapist in Canada. The Alliance, CPA, CUPAC, Toronto

Canadian Association of Occupational Therapists 2002 Profile of occupational therapy practice in Canada. 2nd edn. CAOT, Toronto

Carpenter C 1994 The experience of spinal cord injury: the individual's perspective – implications for rehabilitation practice. Physical Therapy 74(7):614–629

Carpenter C, Hammell KW 2000 Evaluating qualitative research. In: Hammell KW, Carpenter C, Dyck I (eds) Using qualitative research: a practical introduction for occupational and physical therapists. Churchill Livingstone, Edinburgh; pp. 107–119

DeJong G 1979 Independent living: from social movement to analytic paradigm. Archives of Physical Medicine and Rehabilitation 60:435–446

French S, Swain J 1997 Changing disability research: participating and emancipatory research with disabled people. Physiotherapy 83(1):26–32

Glaser B, Strauss A 1967 The discovery of grounded theory. Aldine, Chicago

Goering P, Streiner D 1996 Reconcilable differences: the marriage of qualitative and quantitative methods. Canadian Journal of Psychiatry 41:491–497

Hammell K, Carpenter C 2000 Introduction to qualitative research in occupational and physical therapy. In: Hammell KW, Carpenter C, Dyck I (eds) Using qualitative research: a practical introduction for occupational and physical therapists. Churchill Livingstone, Edinburgh; pp. 1–12

Hollis V, Openshaw S, Goble R 2002 Conducting focus groups: purpose and practicalities. British Journal of Occupational Therapy 65(1):2–8

Krefting L 1991 Rigor in qualitative research: the assessment of trustworthiness. American Journal of Occupational Therapy 45(3):214–222

Krueger R 1994 Focus groups: a practical guide for applied research. 2nd edn. Sage, Thousand Oaks, CA

Law M (ed) 2002 Evidence-based rehabilitation: a guide to practice. Slack, Thorofare, NJ

MacDonald C, Fudge E 2001 Planning and recruiting the sample for focus groups and in-depth interviews. Qualitative Health Research 11(1):117–125

Moore M, Beazley S, Maelzer J 1998 Researching disability issues. Open University Press, Buckingham

Morgan D 1997 Focus groups as qualitative research. 2nd edn. Sage, Thousand Oaks, CA

Morgan D 1998 Practical strategies for combining qualitative and quantitative methods: applications for health research. Qualitative Health Research 8(3):362–376

Oliver M 1993 Re-defining disability: a challenge in research. In: Swain J, Finkelstein V, French S, Oliver M (eds) Disabling barriers: enabling environments. Sage, London; pp. 61–67

Pope C, Mays N (eds) 1999 Qualitative research in health care. 2nd edn. BMJ Books, London

Rebeiro K 2000 Client perspectives on occupational therapy practice: are we truly client-centered? Canadian Journal of Occupational Therapy 65(5):279–285

Ritchie JE 1999 Using qualitative research to enhance the evidence-based practice of health care providers. Australian Journal of Physiotherapy 45:251–256

Sim J, Snell J 1996 Focus groups in physiotherapy evaluation and research. Physiotherapy 82(3):189–198

Sofaer S 1999 Qualitative methods: what are they and why use them? Health Services Research 34(5):1102–1118

Stone E, Priestley M 1996 Parasites, pawns and partners: disability and the role of non-disabled researchers. British Journal of Sociology 47(4):699–716

Williamson C 2001 What does involving consumers in research mean? Quarterly Journal of Medicine (editorial) 94:661–664

Yoshida K, Willi V, Parker I, Self H, Carpenter S, Pfeiffer D 1998 Disability partnerships in research and teaching in Canada and the United States. Physiotherapy Canada Summer:198–205

Zarb G (ed) 1995 Removing disabling barriers. Policy Studies Institute, London

FURTHER READING

Duggan CH, Dijkers M 2001 Quality of life after spinal cord injury: a qualitative study. Rehabilitation Psychology 46(1):3–27

Waterton C, Wynne B 1999 Can focus groups access community views? In: Barbour R, Kitzinger J (eds) Developing focus group research: politics, theory and practice. Sage, Thousand Oaks, CA; pp. 127–142

6

Ensuring a client perspective in evidence-based rehabilitation research

Deborah Corring

OVERVIEW

The following three chapters describe qualitative research designed to generate evidence with which to inform service delivery and modes of practice. Congruent with the participatory approaches to research outlined in the previous chapters, these authors all demonstrate a commitment to client-centred approaches to research. This chapter, by Deborah Corring, discusses research undertaken to address the curious gulf between client-centred research and theories about client-centred practice. Despite espousing a client-centred philosophy, occupational therapists had neglected to seek clients' perspectives concerning what 'client cen-tred' means, or what client-centred practice would look like. A subsequent study explored quality of life issues for both consumers of mental health services and their family members, generating qualitative evidence with which to inform future practice.

K.H.

INTRODUCTION

This chapter describes research that explored how clients define client-centred care and their quality of life issues. The research findings build on and support the assertion that involving clients in decisions concerning their care, and in the evalu-ation of the services they receive, results both in improved outcomes and client satisfaction, and can therefore be considered important evidence on which to base practice (Corring & Cook 1999, Hammell 2001, Law 1998). This chapter further asserts that it is time for rehabilitation profession-als routinely to incorporate clients' perspectives on matters pertaining to their care. It is hoped that this chapter will challenge rehabilitation pro-fessionals to make a fundamental change in their approach to the evaluation of their practice, resulting in an intolerance for any approach that does not include the client perspective.

PERSON-CENTRED CARE: AN EVOLVING INFLUENCE ON THE PRACTICE OF REHABILITATION

One of the most influential elements on the evolution of healthcare services over the past 20 years has been the demand by consumers/clients/patients for a more responsive system of service delivery (Law et al 1995).

The occupational therapy profession has sup-ported a client-centred approach to practice in many important ways, including the development of practice guidelines and recommendations concerning the involvement of clients in the evalu-ation of our services (Canadian Association of Occupational Therapists (CAOT) 1997, CAOT et al 1999). This client-centred approach to practice

has been shown to result in improved client satis-faction and improved outcomes (Law 1998), and can therefore be considered an evidence-based approach to delivering services (Hammell 2001).

There are many complex issues related to a person-centred approach to practice, including: the balance of caring for the client and maintain-ing an appropriate relationship as a caregiver, the practical realities of patient or client involvement in clinical decision-making, the building of a patient–professional partnership that involves empowerment and the sharing of power, and the difficulties in implementing such an approach. The particular difficulties of implementing client-centred practices in institutions dominated by the medical model have been noted by Sumsion (1999).

Despite an espoused client-centred orientation, the rehabilitation professions have rarely under-taken collaborative research or service evaluation partnerships with clients. If congruence is to occur between theory and practice, rehabilitation pro-fessionals need routinely to incorporate the client perspective in research and service evaluation.

WHY IS A CLIENT PERSPECTIVE SO IMPORTANT?

A review of the client satisfaction literature reveals many of the potential benefits of client involvement in evaluation. For at least three decades, research studies have confirmed the effectiveness of including client input in serv-ice delivery evaluation (Corring & Cook 1999, Hart & Bassett 1975). As early as 1960, researchers such as Elling et al (1996), who were researching client satisfaction with services for children being treated for rheumatic fever, began to question why some patients apparently participated at higher levels in programmes than others. They were surprised both by the positive influences of patient understanding of their illness and their proposed treatments and by the effect of sup-portive, positive relationships with clinicians, and increased levels of participation. Research studies have also linked client involvement in goal-setting and decision-making about their health with better outcomes (Foon 1987, Willer & Miller 1978).

Comparison of client and professional opinions and perspectives has also resulted in a few 'surprises' for researchers. Little or no agreement has been found between clients and professionals in basic areas such as preferred approaches to service delivery, expectations of clients, definitions of 'rehabilitation' and 'getting better', priorities of treatment goals and presenting problems, and definitions of leisure (Casier 2001, Hart & Bassett 1975, Mayer & Rosenblatt 1974, Prager & Tanaka 1980). These differences have been noted by researchers for almost 30 years.

It would appear that we no longer need to be surprised about the contributions that a client perspective can bring to our areas of inquiry. Clearly, the rehabilitation professions could benefit from research involving our clients, particularly when addressing issues of evidence-based practice. Once the decision has been made to involve clients in a research endeavour, the choice of research methods must be addressed as an important issue. As many researchers have noted, the choice of research methodology should be informed by the problem it seeks to address. If we are seeking to measure concrete variables, then quantitative methods are clearly appropriate. However, if we wish to know what it means to live with an impairment, what contributes to quality of life, or what makes life meaningful, qualitative methods would be the more effective choice (Hammell & Carpenter 2000). Taking the position that studying phenomena related to human beings is different from investigations in the natural sciences, Slife & Gantt (1999) suggest that it is time for a new level of sophistication. To quote a famous scientist, Albert Einstein, 'not everything that counts can be counted, not everything that can be counted counts'. It would seem apparent that the incorporation of client perspectives requires a qualitative approach to inquiry.

ACQUIRING A CLIENT PERSPECTIVE: MY RESEARCH EXPERIENCES

In order to frame the inquiry and finalize the research design, I began by asking the 'who, what, when, where and why' of it (Box 6.1).

Box 6.1 The who, what, when, where and why?

- *What* is the issue or clinical irritation?
- *When*, *where* and *with whom* can I best explore the issue?
- *What* will, or might I find after I have explored the issue?
- *Why* might the results make a difference to practice and *why* is this important?

THE FIRST RESEARCH PROJECT
What was the issue or clinical irritation?

Several times during my years of practice I experienced what I have come to label 'clinical irritations'. It bothered me, for example, that many clinicians began every interaction with a client with the presumption that the client was unable to provide an accurate description of his or her symptoms, course of illness, effects of the illness on their lives, etc., and that whatever was heard would therefore have to be verified through a more credible, reliable source and/or therapists' 'objective' assessments. I had begun my career some 30 years ago when the 'medical model' was firmly entrenched in the mental health institution where I worked, and persons like myself (a non-physician) were certainly not encouraged to question the 'expert' clinician approach to patient care. It bothered me that maintaining a 'professional distance' apparently meant that I was expected to be careful not to get too close to the person presenting with symptoms of illness. While the concept of professional distance may have some important elements, I saw many of my colleagues withdraw to such a distance that they appeared to lose sight of the person to whom they were ostensibly providing service. It bothered me that we did not take time to get to know the person behind the symptoms – what it was like for them to live with their illnesses, how these affected their sense of self, their family, their dreams, hopes and wishes – as we did with assessing symptoms, deficits in functioning, and what *we* perceived to be their problem areas. Early in my career I found myself seeking out biographies written by people who had experienced severe and persistent mental illnesses, and found these to be important sources of information for understanding what it was like to live with these illnesses.

I embraced with considerable enthusiasm the Canadian Association of Occupational Therapists' *Guidelines for Client-Centred Practice* (1983) when they were published, and have tried to promote their use in my capacity as a clinician and administrator. However, while examining the occupational therapy literature concerning client-centred care many years later, I realized that even though our profession had been discussing this concept since 1983, there were still no reports of client-generated definitions of client-centred care in the occupational therapy literature. I found this both a surprising and a somewhat alarming omission – so alarming that I decided to focus the thesis for my MSc on this area of inquiry. As Hammell (2001) noted, it is ironic that, although occupational therapists have debated this topic for some time, few occupational therapy researchers have sought to explore the meaning to clients of client-centred care. This reality exposes the unstable basis for our claim to client-centred philosophy as a foundation for our practice (Hammell 2001).

When, where and with whom could I best explore this issue?

Deciding on a research plan and choosing an adviser

The two decisions concerning my choice of adviser and client group were relatively easy. I was lucky enough to be associated with an adviser who has considerable experience in the use of qualitative methods. After more than 20 years in the mental health field, I wanted to see whether I could make a difference in the ways in which services were delivered to people living with severe and persistent mental illness.

With the guidance of my supervisor I planned a research study that would employ the qualitative strategies of focus groups (Morgan 1997) and participatory action research (Whyte 1991) to explore a client definition of client-centred care. Participatory action research (PAR) is a powerful design strategy that is client-centred and that focuses on practical problems of importance to the individuals who are the subjects of the study (Whyte 1991). PAR requires an emphasis on learning from participants, valuing their subjective experiences and enabling their participation in the full research process (Rogers & Palmer-Erbs 1994).

I felt the participatory action research approach was of particular importance for my study because I was concerned about the effect that my professional background might have on recruitment of participants, upon participants' feelings of trust and safety, and their willingness to criticize both the services they had received and the professionals who had provided these services over the course of their mental illnesses.

Ensuring participation in the research process

I decided to approach the two facilitators of our institution's patient council to see whether they might be interested in co-investigator roles in the project. Both individuals were enthusiastic, and so began some very exciting discussions regarding who to recruit for the focus groups, where these individuals might best be found, where to hold the groups so that individuals would feel safe when participating in them, what questions needed to be asked and who should facilitate the groups.

Eventually we agreed that we would seek out participants who were members of consumer survivor agencies. These consumer survivor agencies were funded as part of the community investment effort by the Ontario Ministry of Health following the release of the mental health reform policy document *Putting People First* in 1993. The consumer survivor agencies were designed to be staffed by individuals who had personal experience as consumers of the mental health service system and were intended to provide self-help, advocacy and peer support services to individuals currently receiving mental health services. Given their mandate, we thought that this group of individuals might feel more comfortable than current inpatients or registered outpatients of the local institution in an exercise that would potentially include a critique of the service system on which they depended.

We organized our thoughts into a research proposal and an ethics review application for the local university's ethics review board. Once the proposal and ethics had been approved, we began the process of recruitment. The three of us met with the executive directors of two consumer survivor agencies (i.e. agencies run for and by individuals who have used – and in many cases continue to use – formal mental health services). Agreement was reached regarding how volunteers would be approached for the focus groups. One agency decided to put an advertisement in their newsletter and asked us to hold an information session regarding the project. The other put up a poster in its 'drop-in' centre. The first agency also approached individuals directly to determine their willingness to participate. As a result, two groups were conducted with the first agency and one with the second.

The focus groups

Before undertaking the first focus group, the client-researchers and I met to discuss the facilitator and observer roles that we would play, and reviewed Morgan's (1997) recommendations regarding the purpose of focus groups, the role of participants and facilitators, and the strategies that could be used to maximize the effectiveness of these groups. When the time arrived to do the first focus group, we were ready. We had arrived early in order to set up the audiotaping equipment and the room. We met with each potential participant to review the letter of information regarding the project and ensure that they understood and were comfortable with the expectations – including audiotaping of the group. We asked them to sign the consent form if they were willing to proceed; all of those who were approached agreed to participate.

The group began with introductions of the two facilitators and their backgrounds, as well as my own as the observer. The purpose of the focus group was repeated, and a description of the roles that the facilitators and the observer would play was provided. The interview guide that we used is illustrated in Box 6.2.

The group began slowly but warmed up after about 10 minutes. Client-centred care was not a

---

Box 6.2 Focus group questions

- What does client-centred care mean to you? How would you describe it?
- If mental health services revolved around you and your needs, what would they look like?
- What sort of things in a hospital or community agency help or hinder a person with your kind of needs to achieve their goals in life?
- If you were asked by people who decide what and how mental health services are provided to you as a client of those services, what would you suggest is the number one priority they should address?

---

familiar term to group members and this prompted a discussion among the participants as to what it might mean. This quickly prompted each member of the group to describe at length their personal experience in dealing with the healthcare and social service systems over the duration of their illness. For many people this spanned two or three decades. As the observer, I found these accounts very moving. I had a sense of wonderment and admiration for these individuals who had maintained a sense of themselves and demonstrated such caring for their peers while managing such demanding illnesses. Further, I felt a sense of embarrassment at being associated with what they described as an uncaring, unhelpful service system. The group lasted for 2 hours and, even though the focus group interview guide contained probes to prompt exploration of client-centred care, discussion regarding client-centred care had been relatively brief and near the end of the session. This made me wonder what had gone wrong. Why hadn't we discussed elements of client-centred care?

In an effort to ensure trustworthiness in this research, I transcribed the first group's conversations so that my adviser could review these and provide feedback regarding such issues as how the group was facilitated, how we might concentrate in future groups on areas that we might have missed, and whether any questions needed to be added or modified. I was concerned that the group had been a failure and that not much of anything had focused on what I wanted to know.

Dr Cook explained that there is no such thing as a total failure: qualitative researchers seek to explore what participants have to say about a phenomenon and to understand *their* priorities and perspectives. There are no right or wrong answers. The task of the researcher is to listen, probe where necessary to ensure understanding, transcribe verbatim what has been said, and then set about organizing what has been said into themes utilizing a coding system. She encouraged us to begin the next group with an invitation to take a few minutes to discuss and understand what client-centred care meant to the participants, and then continue the discussion to get a detailed elaboration of what participants thought client-centred care might actually look like when receiving services from professionals. This was effective advice. The second group had no difficulty staying on topic and engaged in an hour and a half of active discussion about what client-centred care should look like if one received services in that fashion. The third group also focused early in the discussion and spent an hour and a half in conversation. Reviews of transcripts from the three groups by myself, the co-investigators and adviser resulted in agreement that we had reached 'data saturation'. Saturation refers to the point at which an investigator has obtained sufficient data to feel confident that an understanding of the phenomenon has been achieved (DePoy & Gitlin 1994). Morgan (1997) suggests that saturation is usually reached after three or four focus groups, and occurs when 'additional data collection no longer generates new understanding' (p. 43). This meant it was time for analysis.

Analysing the data

Analysis of data in qualitative research is a very different experience to that in quantitative research. It is a labour-intensive process of repeatedly reviewing the transcripts and continuously contrasting and comparing what has been said so that themes, categories and other levels of understanding can be gleaned from the data. Because this was a student project, I produced a preliminary analysis for discussion with my adviser and the co-investigators. After they had vetted it,

we took it back to a number of the focus group participants for member checking as another way of ensuring trustworthiness. The changes made by the clients included: altering the word 'professional' to 'service provider' to reflect better their experiences in both healthcare and social service agencies; the renaming of an element from 'apathy' to 'disillusionment'; and the addition of three elements – negative effect on the healing process, meeting their own needs, and laws.

Findings of the study

This research generated the first client definition of client-centred care to be described in the occupational therapy literature (Corring & Cook 1999). Findings were organized under two main themes: the client in the client–service provider relationship and the client in the social and mental health system. Under each theme three categories were identified – what's wrong, the effect on the client, and what's needed. Elements under each category varied in number from three to seven, and also varied in content. Examples of *what's wrong* in the *client–service provider relationship* were elements such as 'negative attitudes' and 'indifference to patients as fellow human beings'. Included in the *effect on client* were elements such as 'fear' and 'disillusionment', and within *what's needed* were elements such as 'value the client' and 'need for common ground'.

Under the second theme – *the client in the social and mental health system* – the categories of *what's wrong* included 'service providers not being accountable' and 'stigma'; the *effect on the client* included elements of being 'marginalized' and 'not a societal priority'. Finally, under *what's needed*, 'peer support services' and 'clients involved in making change' were listed. Under the general theme of 'valuing of the client as a human being', the participants had identified 11 key concepts of client-centred care (Box 6.3).

The findings of this study also contain several important messages. Perhaps the most poignant is the impassioned plea from clients for service providers – and society in general – to recognize their human strengths and frailties and to value them as they would any other human

Box 6.3 Eleven key concepts of caring

1. The adoption of a positive, caring and welcoming attitude towards clients
2. The development of full relationships with clients
3. The finding of common ground with clients
4. The assurance of informed decision-making for clients
5. The facilitation of healing and recovery
6. The use of clients in the education of professionals
7. An intolerance for stereotyping and stigmatizing attitudes of professionals
8. Assurance of accountability of professionals to clients
9. Education of the general public
10. Valuing of the benefits of self-help services
11. Advocating for laws that will protect vulnerable individuals

system that provides mental health clients 'with more meaning, more purpose, more success and more satisfaction with their lives' (Anthony 1993, p. 16). As a well known occupational therapist, Elizabeth Yerxa (1980) said over two decades ago: 'our profession in the future should be evaluated not only on the basis of measurable, scientific outcomes, but also by what it contributes to the individual's human dignity, sense of mastery and self respect' (p. 534).

However, this study also illustrated that a caring relationship between clients and service providers, while critical, is insufficient without other social and system changes. Occupational therapists must advocate a service delivery system that is more humane, more focused on recovery and more responsive to client needs. We cannot just sit on the sidelines and espouse client-centred care: we must make it happen.

THE SECOND RESEARCH PROJECT

My second venture into qualitative research happened 2 years after completion of my Master's degree, when I decided to determine whether there was any interest among service agencies in utilizing evaluation strategies that would not only include but emphasize client input. After contact with several agencies I received an inquiry regarding a potential project from a local health council representative. They asked whether I would work with a consumer survivor agency (i.e. run for and by individuals who have received or are receiving services from the mental health service system) in a funded project that it was hoped would focus on client satisfaction with local mental health service providers.

Gaining access and agreement on the research question

I arranged to meet with the executive director and two other people from the consumer survivor agency to plan the details of how we would proceed and to ensure that the focus of the enquiry would be of importance to them. Recognizing their role as co-investigators in the participatory action research framework meant a discussion of what

being. The ubiquity with which phrases involving the recognition of their worth as human beings occurred in the transcripts is illustrated by the following excerpts:

'they're [the clients] considered to be less than human ...'

'I want some kind of response – an emotional response, that I exist as a human being.'

'We should be appreciated for the person, people that we are.'

The participants provided support for occupational therapy's contention that 'every person has intrinsic dignity and worth' (CAOT 1997, p. 31). Sadly, service provision clearly failed to reflect this philosophy.

How might these findings impact on practice and why are they important?

The findings of this study suggest that mental health service providers (including occupational therapists) must work actively towards establishing common ground with clients. Clients need to be viewed as experts concerning their own life experiences, aspirations and life goals. Empowerment and advocacy are critical to recovery, and accountability to clients should be understood and made transparent by all professionals. Together we must strive to achieve a mental health service the focus of the inquiry should be, how and where we would recruit individuals to be part of focus groups, and what roles they would play in the research process. We parted with what I thought was a well developed plan and a date for my return to do the first focus group. I arrived on the designated date, did some preliminary training with the woman who was to be my co-facilitator, set up the tape recorder, welcomed and oriented the participants to the process, and obtained their consent. The first focus group went well and we made plans for a second group, but before the second group could take place the project hit a snag.

The executive director called to explain that when she had reported on our progress at the last health council committee meeting a number of problems had been raised by other committee members. Local service providers were not interested in an evaluation of their services, and representatives from the family support group felt that funding for the project had been intended for both themselves and the consumer group. The executive director and I agreed to meet with representatives of the service providers, family support group and the health council to see whether we could work out a plan that all stakeholders would be able to support.

After a lengthy discussion, it was agreed to proceed with a plan that would explore quality of life issues for both consumers of mental health services and their family members. The focus on quality of life as an area of exploration was emphasized as an area of importance by both the consumer and family group. It was hoped that the results of such an exploration could be used in influencing funding from the Ministry of Health.

It was agreed that three focus groups would be conducted with consumers and three with family members. Congruent with the principles of participatory action research, the interview guide would be developed collaboratively in order to ensure the focus of inquiry was one that was important to each group. Further, each focus group would be facilitated by myself and a co-facilitator from their peer group, preliminary analysis of themes would be member checked by representatives of both groups, and the final analysis of data would also be developed collaboratively.

How, when and where would the data be collected?

In a format similar to that of the first research project, it was agreed that the best way to recruit participants would be through their respective support groups. The family support group also chose to take advantage of a local journalist's offer to do a feature article on their efforts and include a call for focus group participants as part of the coverage. It was further decided to hold the focus groups in the familiar settings of their support group locations. Focus groups for clients took place during the day at a time convenient to participants, and the family groups took place in the evenings.

What did we find out?

Client perspectives centred around two themes: 'peer support and advocacy' and 'elements essential to successful recovery'. The first theme consisted of three categories – needing a place to belong, a place to help others or to help yourself, and a continued need for advocacy. The second theme consisted of nine categories, labelled as follows: needing a good support system to maintain health, needing to feel worthwhile, financial security facilitates recovery, need to increase understanding of illness, recognize our need to care for our children, need to be part of the community, need for personal living space, need a positive attitude, and need time for recovery. The following excerpts from the transcripts illustrate some of what clients had to say.

Several client participants described their consumer survivor agency as a place where they felt safe, where all were created equal, where they could be with friends who became like family to them and where they could have fun:

'I call this group a family. It's my family, and if I need help – if it's [the illness] going to happen again – the only place I'm going to go is here …'

Several participants spoke of the importance of caring for and helping others, and the positive effects that this has had on their own self-esteem. Involvement in peer support allowed them to learn from others and to share what they had learned from their own life experiences:

'I try to get into the community and do volunteering and pick up my self-esteem, and feel good about myself … when I'm helping people I feel good.'

Positive, caring attitudes of families, friends and service providers were described as critical factors in regaining and maintaining health and quality of life. People who would listen and provide support, understand and provide validation of oneself, who could be trusted and who would do more than just 'tolerate you' were important to all group members:

'I would think quality of life is having a … when one has a mental disability, its having good supports to help you through the rough times, a good support system.'

When clients were asked how they spent their leisure time, many commented that free time was one thing they had too much of and that they would much rather have an opportunity to work. They talked about the importance of work. They talked of the difficulties of finding employment and the paradox of disability pensions. Many saw employment as closely tied to an improved quality of life and wished that greater opportunities to work were available.

Clients feel they are often placed in a position of begging and of being forced to choose between what service providers describe as 'luxuries' – such as a phone, food or cable television. They are limited in their ability to join in community activities owing to limited funds. Many connected their perpetual worries about money and bills to a slowed recovery from illness. Many also felt that they had been forced into conforming to the stereotype of a mental health consumer – that of a lazy person content to sit on welfare – when they perceived themselves as being trapped by the 'system'.

Being a parent is always challenging. There are substantial, additional challenges to raising a child for someone who is also struggling with a mental illness, the stigma that is attached to that illness and the financial dilemmas that accompany unemployment. People also indicated the desire to ensure that their children would not endure the hardships that they did as children:

'I ask forgiveness, especially from my younger daughter because I was not there for her when I was sick – she was only a few months old …'

Expectations by society, service providers and colleagues that individuals with mental illness will have a speedy recovery sometimes place these individuals in precarious situations:

'I had a new job, I was being rushed from place to place, and I had deadlines, deadlines, deadlines. The husband was coming back home, the kids were here, all the normal stuff that people with healthy minds can go through – and you don't have a healthy mind, you can't go through everything as fast as everybody else … that affects your quality of life because everybody expects me to be first.'

In summary, concrete indicators for improved quality of life for clients include continued and improved peer support and self-help activities, and a health system that promotes the necessary elements for recovery outlined in this study. It would appear that significant investment in these two areas would have a resulting positive effect on quality of life for mental health clients.

Family perspectives were organized under one primary theme: 'their quality of life is our quality of life'. This consisted of the following nine categories: we're the bottom line; you learn to live with a stranger; you live with constant uncertainty; support for consumers improves quality of life for families; families need supports too; people just don't understand or don't want to understand; planning for when I'm gone; taking time out for yourself; and laws and legislation.

Family members spoke of the 24-hour-a-day job they encounter when their relatives are ill. Normal family roles and activities are put on hold while the family is consumed by caring for their loved one. Being a constant caregiver is draining, leaving no time for enjoyment of life or leisure. Family members pick up the pieces when all else fails, and find that their ability to cope decreases with age and their own compromised physical and emotional health:

'I guess the best is to say you exist, it's not a quality of life, it's an existence. You go to bed at night with one ear to the phone, you get up in the morning hoping that it won't ring, and if it don't ring you worry how come, and it affects your whole family … it's a 24-hour-a-day job.'

Family members talked of the strained, 'on edge' relationships they had with their relatives. They talked of the difficulties of feeling rejected, being lied to and lied about, treated badly, and of often feeling that their child was no longer the child whom they had raised. Overwhelming frustration and fear were expressed by many family members as they struggled with questions about their relative, such as: When will they get sick again? How much do you have to accept? How much can you hope for and what does the future hold?

Family members agreed that if their relative was well supported with services in the community, the family's emotional load was significantly decreased. Families are struggling with the burden of these illnesses with little apparent recognition by the mental health system of their need for counselling, education, support, recognition, advocacy, financial assistance or for partnerships with mental health professionals.

Caregivers have found they must make time to focus on their own needs, find relief from the overwhelming stress, and find periods of peace and tranquillity at home. They find joy in small things, spend time with remaining friends and consciously seek enjoyment:

'One of the psychiatrists lately was the first one (after 21 years), he took me by the arm and explained to me that I had to start to look after myself … [he said] "we deal with all the Pauls, the Davids, the Elizabeths during the day, but when you have the person at home you're dealing with it 24 hours a day. We can walk away, we can go home, we can sleep, we can enjoy a meal, but you people can't …".'

In summary, concrete indicators for improved quality of life for family members are based in a mental health system that ensures support programmes, help when needed, and education in a responsive and helpful fashion. Significant investment in these areas will potentially improve quality of life for both family members and their ill

relatives and, as a result, prevent family members from becoming ill themselves.

How might these results impact on practice and why are they important?

'Empowerment is a little like obscenity; you have trouble defining it, but you know it when you see it' (Temkin et al 1995, p. 4). The message regarding empowerment rang out loud and clear in the comments of clients in the focus groups. They need professionals to respect and support their efforts at self-help and peer support, and to acknowledge these as complementary services in a continuum of available services.

The factors identified as elements associated with successful recovery deserve particular attention by professionals. Recovery is a relatively new consideration for individuals with severe and persistent mental illness. The *World Health Report on Mental Health* (World Health Organization 2001) estimates that up to 77% of persons with schizophrenia can live without relapses, but only 35% of people seek help even when care is available and affordable. The effects of stigma and lack of public education are still powerful barriers to recovery, yet achieving recovery appears to be a concrete indicator of quality of life for clients. Recovery is aided by an effective support system, recognition of the importance of work and financial security, allowing sufficient time to deal with the experience of severe trauma, regaining a place in the community, regaining a positive sense of self, and injecting a sense of hope in overcoming the challenges of a devastating illness.

Family members talked extensively of the interweaving of the illness experience of the mentally ill family member with the overall functioning of the family. Repeatedly, family members talked of the 24-hour nature of their task and the unremitting stress that a family member's illness places on the family because of the constant uncertainty, stigma, lack of understanding and lack of assistance they receive with their struggle to cope with the situation. Their experiences have highlighted for them the services they and their relatives require for the future. Services that will support, educate and involve family members as well as clients are likely to improve the quality of life for families of people with mental illness. Continued development of family support programmes, true partnerships with professionals, back-up crisis and medical services that families can count on, and education for families regarding the illness, its treatment and hopes for the future would have profound effects on a family's quality of life.

CONCLUDING THOUGHTS

Let me end by emphasizing what was said in the introduction: it is time for occupational therapists to exhibit congruence between theory and practice. We cannot say we are client-centred if we routinely leave the client's perspective out of inquiries into the effectiveness of our practices, and out of the inquiries that build or reaffirm the theoretical basis of our profession. We can no longer be surprised that client involvement in these activities can teach us something; the value of client involvement has been demonstrated for at least 30 years. It is time for occupational therapists to show no shame in caring for the individual to whom they deliver service, to value clients' lived experiences, to ensure that clients' goals are what professionals seek to support, and to ensure that clients are treated like valuable human beings. It is time for occupational therapists and other rehabilitation professionals to help build a service system that helps clients and their families to attain a quality of life that is satisfying and fulfilling. Ensuring a client perspective in evidence-based rehabilitation research will go a long way to achieving this timely objective.

ACKNOWLEDGEMENTS

Joanne Valiant Cook, the person who has guided me throughout my MSc and PhD research, is one of the pioneers of qualitative research in occupational therapy. She has made my life richer by sharing her love of qualitative research with me. She is a tireless and supportive adviser whom I can't thank enough for the gift of her knowledge and insights.

REFERENCES

Anthony W 1993 Recovery from mental illness: a guiding vision of the mental health system in the 1990s. Psychosocial Rehabilitation Journal 16:11–23

Canadian Association of Occupational Therapists, Health and Welfare Canada 1983 Guidelines for the client-centred practice of occupational therapy. Department of National Health and Welfare, Ottawa

Canadian Association of Occupational Therapists 1997 Enabling occupation: an occupational therapy perspective. CAOT, Ottawa

Canadian Association of Occupational Therapists, Association of Canadian Occupational Therapy University Programmes, Association of Canadian Regulatory Organizations and Presidents' Advisory Committee 1999 Joint position statement on evidence based occupational therapy. Canadian Journal of Occupational Therapy 66(5):267–269

Casier S 2001 Leisure from the client's perspective: when do you have too much? Master of Clinical Science thesis, University of Western Ontario, London, Ontario

Corring D, Cook JV 1999 Client centred care means that I am a valued human being. Canadian Journal of Occupational Therapy 66:71–82

DePoy E, Gitlin LN 1994 Introduction to research: multiple strategies for health and human services. Mosby, St Louis

Elling R, Whitmore R, Green M 1996 Patient participation in a paediatric program. Journal of Health and Human Behaviour 1:183–191

Foon AE 1987 Locus of control as a predictor of psychotherapy. British Journal of Medical Psychology 60:99–107

Hammell KW 2001 Using qualitative research to inform the client-centred evidence-based practice of occupational therapy. British Journal of Occupational Therapy 64(5):228–234

Hammell K, Carpenter C 2000 Introduction to qualitative research in occupational and physical therapy. In: Hammell K, Carpenter C, Dyck I (eds) Using qualitative research: a practical introduction for occupational and physical therapists. Churchill Livingstone, Edinburgh; pp. 1–12

Hart WT, Bassett L 1975 Measuring consumer satisfaction in a mental health centre. Hospital and Community Psychiatry 26(8):512–515

Law M 1998 Does client-centred care make a difference? In: Law M (ed) Client-centred occupational therapy. Slack, New Jersey; pp. 19–27

Law M, Baptiste S, Mills J 1995 Client-centred practice: what does it mean and does it make a difference? Canadian Journal of Occupational Therapy 62:250–257

Mayer JE, Rosenblatt 1974 Clash in perspectives between mental patients and staff. American Journal of Orthopsychiatry 44:432–441

Morgan D 1997 Focus groups as qualitative research. Sage, Thousand Oaks, CA

Ontario Ministry of Health 1993 Putting people first: the reform of mental health services in Ontario. Queen's Printer for Ontario, Toronto

Prager E, Tanaka H 1980 Self-assessment: the client's perspective. Social Work January:32–35

Rogers SE, Palmer-Erbs V 1994 Participatory action research: implications for research and evaluation in psychiatric rehabilitation. Psychosocial Rehabilitation Journal 18(2):3–12

Slife BD, Gantt EE 1999 Methodological pluralism: a framework for psychotherapy research. Journal of Clinical Psychology 55:1453–1465

Sumsion T (ed) 1999 Client-centred practice in occupational therapy: a guide to implementation. Churchill Livingstone, London

Temkin T, Silverman C, Segal SP 1995 Making self help work. Journal of the California Alliance of the Mentally Ill 6:4–5

Whyte WF (ed) 1991 Participatory action research. Sage, Newbury Park, CA

Willer B, Miller GH 1978 On the relationship of client satisfaction to client characteristics and outcome of treatment. Journal of Clinical Psychology 34(1):157–160

World Health Organization 2001 World Health Report 2001: mental health: new understanding, new hope. WHO, Geneva

Yerxa EJ 1980 Occupational therapy's role in creating a future climate of caring. American Journal of Occupational Therapy 34:529–534

FURTHER READING

Corring D 2002 Quality of life: perspectives of people with mental illnesses and family members. Psychiatric Rehabilitation Journal 25(4):350–358

Prince PN, Prince CR 2001 Subjective quality of life in the evaluation of programs for people with serious and persistent mental illness. Clinical Psychology Review 21(7):1005–1036

Rogers SE, Palmer-Erbs V 1994 Participatory action research: implications for research and evaluation in psychiatric rehabilitation. Psychosocial Rehabilitation Journal 18(2):3–12

Wolf J, Boevink W 1999 Mapping the quality of life of people with severe and enduring mental health problems. Mental Health Care 21(7):228–231

7

Integrating grounded theory and action research to develop guidelines for sensitive practice with survivors of childhood sexual abuse

Candice L. Schachter   *Eli Teram*   *Carol A. Stalker*

KEY POINTS

action research; client-centred practice; physical therapy practice; sexual abuse survivors; using research evidence to develop practice guidelines

OVERVIEW

Continuing the theme of generating qualitative evidence to inform modes of practice and service delivery, Candice L. Schachter, Eli Teram and Carol A. Stalker describe research that arose from the healthcare experiences of women survivors of childhood sexual abuse. Committed not solely to undertaking research to explore women survivors' reactions to physical therapy, but to generating guidelines for sensitive practice for healthcare professionals, the researchers demonstrated the fit between client-centred philosophy and action research. The findings of the study, and the process of consultation required to develop the practice guidelines, prompted the researchers to create a handbook that reflected these findings and that is currently in use in clinical education. This chapter demonstrates the translation of research into both education and practice.

K.H.

INTRODUCTION

We undertook a study with three primary goals: (1) to explore women survivors' reactions to physical therapy and their ideas about physical therapy practice that would be sensitive to their needs; (2) to consult with survivors, physical therapists and mental health professionals to develop guidelines for clinicians working unknowingly and knowingly with women survivors of childhood sexual abuse; and (3) to create a handbook that reflected these findings for use in undergraduate and postgraduate clinical education. In this chapter we describe the research process, present highlights of the findings and explore ways that this research can contribute to evidence-based clinical practice.

WHAT PROMPTED THE RESEARCH?

Between 1990 and 1994, one of the authors (C.L.S.) worked as a volunteer co-facilitator of support groups for women survivors of childhood sexual abuse at a sexual assault centre in Ontario. In the spirit of facilitating both care and broader community for women survivors (which included mental health professionals and lay volunteers), Candice worked with a counsellor who was the professional co-facilitator of the groups. Over the 4 years, women survivors in a series of support groups met on a weekly basis. At times, women spoke about their difficulties with health professionals. Some told the group about extreme discomfort that resulted from their interactions with

healthcare providers. One woman described her distress when being examined after a back injury. She said that in a large open-plan clinic, in the presence of many other clinicians and clients, the physical therapist exposed part of her back by a sudden rearrangement of her T-shirt and shorts, without prior consultation or consent. She went on to tell the group that the experience was so disturbing that she could not return to therapy for her severe back pain. Candice's experiences with the groups led her to believe that health professionals could benefit from learning about childhood sexual abuse and other forms of violence, and that this knowledge could help them to work more sensitively with those who had experienced violence.

As a physical therapist who had worked primarily with scientific research methods that focused on physical function, Candice realized that the exploration of these ideas required partnership with people who have expertise related to qualitative research methods and to childhood sexual abuse survivors. The second author (E.T.), who is an experienced qualitative researcher with an interest in the relationship between clients and professionals, offered his methodological expertise for this exploration. The third author (C.A.S.) brought to the project her clinical expertise with childhood sexual abuse survivors. Collaborating on the study described in this chapter has been an exciting way to explore the research questions from a number of perspectives. We have worked together to bring the powerful words of survivors to health professionals, combining survivors' experiences and ideas with the clinical wisdom of practitioners to weave the principles and guidelines of practice that are sensitive to survivors.

To support the rationale for our study, it is necessary to examine the definitions, prevalence rates and empirical findings regarding long-term effects of childhood sexual abuse.

Sexual abuse of children is a covert and criminal activity that is traumatic to the victims. While the term 'child sexual abuse' has been used to describe a wide variety of experiences, the legal and research definitions require two elements: (1) 'sexual activities involving a child, and (2) an "abusive condition" such as coercion or a large age gap between the participants, indicating lack of consensuality' (Finkelhor 1994, p. 32). Sexual activities involving a child are those that the perpetrator performs for his or her sexual stimulation. Abusive conditions have been defined as existing when the perpetrator is significantly older or more mature, when he or she is in a position of power or in a caretaking relationship with the child, or when force, coercion or trickery is used to obtain the child's cooperation (Finkelhor 1994).

The covert and criminal nature of child sexual abuse does not allow us to know its actual incidence, as statistics can report only the number of cases reported to child welfare or police officials. We can, however, estimate the prevalence of child sexual abuse from adult retrospective surveys. Because of differences in the definitions of child sexual abuse used, the age used to define the end of childhood (16 or 18 years) and the populations studied, the prevalence rates vary greatly from study to study. Nevertheless, Finkelhor (1994) concluded that 'enough credible figures cluster around or exceed 20% to suggest that the number of female victims has been at least this high' (p. 37). The same review concluded that a conservative estimate of the prevalence of rates for men would be 5–10%.

A number of studies have reported an association between child sexual abuse and a range of medical conditions. A history of child sexual abuse has been found to be more prevalent, compared with comparison groups, in a variety of clinical samples including those with chronic pelvic pain, gastrointestinal disorders, irritable bowel syndrome and recurrent headaches (e.g. Felitti 1991, Harrop-Griffeths et al 1988, Reiter & Gambone 1990, Walker et al 1993). Others have reported that, compared with non-abused controls, survivors of child sexual abuse have a higher prevalence of medical problems, somatization, health risk behaviours, family physician visits, hospitalizations and surgeries (Finestone et al 2000, Lechner et al 1993, Springs & Friedrich 1992).

Some authors have pointed out that this research suffers from methodological problems (Fry 1993, Laws 1993). However, after a rigorous critique of a number of studies, Fry (1993) concluded that there are recurring themes in the research 'to do with child sexual abuse and later "nonpsychological" consequences ... in the areas of somatic anxiety ... and health-care utilization associated with a range of physical symptoms' (p. 99). Fry's argument is that the research demonstrates that child sexual abuse is frequently found in combination with a history of child physical and emotional abuse, neglect and a variety of dysfunctional family dynamics. He suggests that it might be more accurate to consider child sexual abuse to be a 'marker' of more general child neglect, which appears to constitute a serious risk factor for a variety of later physical and psychological health problems.

The prevalence rates of child sexual abuse in combination with the evidence that women survivors have greater numbers of health problems suggests that health professionals work with survivors on a frequent basis. Historically, physical therapy education has not examined the implications of this conclusion. The core curriculum used in Canada has focused on musculoskeletal, cardiorespiratory and neuromuscular assessment and treatment in order to prepare the student for entry-level physical therapy practice. Although the curriculum has traditionally recognized the potential impact of psychosocial issues on clients' lives, the focus has been on the somatic aspects. Our collective experience led us to believe that survivors often experienced difficulty in interactions with health professionals and would welcome opportunities to work with health professionals who had a greater understanding of the effects of trauma and who were willing to work cooperatively with survivors.

Because of the similarities between long-term effects of abuse in women and men, we suspected that men survivors might also experience difficulties with health professionals. We chose to focus on the issues for women survivors for two main reasons. First, prevalence rates are greater for females than for males. Second, there are fewer services for male survivors in Canada, so recruitment of men survivors needed to be directed primarily at cities with agencies that offered services to men survivors. We have now completed interviews with men survivors and are currently analysing the interview transcripts.

CHOOSING THE RESEARCH METHOD

We chose to use grounded theory (Glaser & Strauss 1967) and action research (Reason 1988, 1994) methodologies in this multi-phased work. The first phase centred around interviews with survivors. Participants were recruited through posters and letters sent to agencies, groups and individuals that provide counselling and support for survivors in Saskatoon, Saskatchewan, and in London, Guelph, Kitchener and Waterloo, Ontario. Survivors who were interested in participating in the study contacted the researchers. In order to participate in this study, women were required to have either formal or informal support around issues of sexual abuse, through, for example, counselling or self-help groups. In this way, each participant was able to contact someone within her support system to discuss any issues that arose from the interview.

We interviewed 27 women from Saskatchewan and Ontario who were survivors of child sexual and ritual abuse, and who had received physical therapy treatment or who had considered seeking physical therapy treatment upon referral. Participants signed informed consents and were offered $20 honoraria for their participation in interviews of approximately 60 minutes in length. Two authors (C.L.S. and C.A.S.) conducted the interviews, which were audiotaped and transcribed. Following the conventions of grounded theory research, no attempt was made to predefine what were relevant data or to use predetermined questions. Thus, each interview was very different, as we followed the issues raised by each participant. The focus of each interview, however, was on the experiences, emotions and concerns related to contact with physical therapists and other health professionals. Following the conventions of qualitative research methods, recruitment of new participants ended when the researchers identified saturation of the data (that is, when themes continued to be repeated and no new themes emerged).

The mean age of the participants in phase one was 39 years (range 19–62 years). One woman identified herself as Metis; 26 participants self-identified as Caucasian. The types of conditions for which physical therapy care was sought by the participants were primarily musculoskeletal, carried out in outpatient, inpatient and home-based settings. A small number of participants had also seen physical therapists for cardiorespiratory conditions in home-based settings and inpatient facilities. No participants reported seeing physical therapists for neurological conditions. Conditions included asthma, fractures and sprains, back pain, headaches, neck pain and total joint replacements. Four participants had chosen, after referral, not to see a physical therapist.

Using the constant comparative method (Glaser & Strauss 1967), the data analysis began when the data collection commenced and informed the ongoing interviewing process. Patterns emerging from the data were used to form a substantive theory that encompassed survivors' experiences and ideas for sensitive practices. Using Folio Views 3.1 Infobase Management Software (The Fien Group, Encino, CA, USA), the data were analysed independently by each author and then discussed by us as a group. Although there were variations in the labelling of some categories, there was a consensus regarding the main emerging themes.

Our interpretation of the data was shared with the participants to ensure it reflected their reality – each participant received a copy and was invited to respond. We further confirmed the trustworthiness, credibility and transferability of the analysis and the theory generated in the second and final phases of this study through the feedback of participants and survivors who had not been part of the interview process.

In the second phase of the project, physical therapists and survivors met together in groups on a monthly basis for approximately 6 months to transform the summary and analysis of interviews into more concrete suggestions and guidelines for sensitive practice. The physical therapists in the groups applied the ideas generated from the discussions in their clinical practice and offered feedback to the groups. The groups then used this feedback to refine their recommendations. The information from the interviews and two working groups was used to create the first draft of the *Handbook on Sensitive Practice*.

Phase three entailed a broad consultive process on successive drafts of the handbook. Written comments regarding the first draft were solicited from all individuals who had participated in phases one and two. After incorporating this initial feedback, the second draft was sent to survivors not involved in interviews, counsellors working with survivors and physical therapy clinicians, academics, professional associations and regulatory bodies across Canada. This feedback was incorporated into a third draft which was used as a subject for discussion by physical therapists and physical therapy students in focus groups across Canada. The feedback from these focus groups was used to produce the final version of the Handbook. This broad consultative process was designed to ensure the clinical applicability of the Handbook.

HIGHLIGHTS OF THE FINDINGS

While we set out to explore survivors' experiences of physical therapy and ideas about clinical physical therapy practice that would be sensitive to their needs as survivors, participants spoke not only about physical therapy but about other health professions as well. It was clear from the outset that the ideas women were sharing with us about practice that would be sensitive to their needs as survivors applied to all health professionals and to most circumstances and practice settings.

The reader will note that we use feminine pronouns to refer to the survivor. While our ongoing research is now focused on the experiences of men survivors with health professionals, these ideas have not yet been integrated into the findings reported below.

Ways that long-term effects of abuse may be manifested when seeing a health professional

Participants described a number of feelings and reactions that may be seen as ways that long-term effects of abuse and neglect were manifested during examination and treatment. Many spoke about fear and distrust of the clinician. Many women discussed physical pain that was both a component of the problem for which she was seeking treatment and also cognitively associated with past abuse. Survivors also stressed the need to feel 'in control' – a need that they connected to past violation.

The participants spoke about a number of attitudes and behaviours that they also related to past abuse. For example, many felt ambivalence about their bodies, describing feelings of hate or shame or of disconnection from their bodies. Some reflected on the subsequent conflict between their need to seek treatment for a physical problem and difficulty in caring for their bodies. One woman explained this by saying:

'And [the amount of attention that I give to my body] ebbs and flows too, depending on where I'm at and how well I'm choosing to take care of my body. Which is a very difficult thing for me physically to do, because when you don't live there, it's just sort of a vehicle to get around.'

Most women said that some parts of their examination or treatment 'triggered' or precipitated flashbacks (experiences of reliving a component of past abuse), dissociation or overwhelming emotions such as fear, anxiety, grief or anger. Many survivors also described difficulty expressing their needs in treatment that had apparently developed from their conditioning to be passive as children:

'[The physical therapist did something and] I really freaked but … I didn't show her I was freaking, because our history is that you don't let on if things are a problem for you. You just deal with it however you can … by dissociating or what have you.'

Feeling safe: the most crucial element

The participants repeatedly identified that feeling safe was of crucial importance for them during treatment by any health professional. Aspects of the survivor's current life that evoke memories of her experiences of violation of body, boundaries and trust reinforce her need to seek safety in the present. Feeling safe was linked to treatment adherence and treatment effectiveness. Some women said that if they did not feel safe they could not even remain in treatment. Others indicated that they felt their progress in treatment was seriously hampered if they did not feel safe. Here is one woman's account of her realization:

'I now am beginning to understand that my physical wellness is really very connected to my emotional state, and if I'm not comfortable, if I'm feeling unsafe, then I'm not going to progress as quickly as a physiotherapist would want me to.'

Principles of sensitive practice

Considering safety as the most crucial element for the survivor during treatment, participants identified a number of constructs that could facilitate the feeling of safety that we came to call the 'Principles of Sensitive Practice', summarized in Box 7.1. Participants helped us to envisage the feeling of safety as a 'protective umbrella' for the survivor, with the principles of sensitive practice as the spokes that keep the umbrella of safety open, thus allowing the survivor to participate in the treatment at hand.

Respect

The survivors we spoke with pointed out that, as a result of past abuse during which they were not respected in a fundamental way, they were very sensitive to any hint of disrespect:

'I find [physical therapists and other health professionals] ... don't even consider the fact that maybe you might feel uncomfortable ... A lot of them ... say, "Oh, we just see you as a patient ... we don't see you as a person" ... part of me says, "No, I don't think so! You're human, and I'm human, and [therapy] is a personal thing ... You're looking at my

body, you're touching *my* body and you're asking me about *my* life." *That's personal!*'

Rapport

Establishing and maintaining a positive rapport with the client is critical to her feelings of safety with the clinician. This process must begin at the first moment of clinician–client interaction and be given ongoing attention. The balance of professionalism and friendliness that contributes to positive rapport is partly a function of individual style. However, the clinician who is distant and cold in his or her professionalism is not likely to facilitate a positive connection with the client. Conversely, an overly familiar style can feel invasive and disrespectful. Developing an appropriate balance is crucial, so that the clinician conveys genuine caring while maintaining appropriate boundaries.

Sharing control

As a child, the survivor was not allowed control over her own body. Consequently, in adulthood, the sense of having control is of paramount importance. By sharing control, the client can become a respected, active participant rather than a bystander during treatment. The clinician can seek to work with, rather than on, the client. One woman spoke about her vision of a respectful, cooperative therapeutic relationship with a physical therapist:

'... [the physical therapist] brings definite knowledge and expertise [into treatment] ... I don't know exactly what it is ... it's what her training is about. So, together with what I know and what I can tell her, I would hope that she would be able to ... assess the situation and offer alternatives ... So, instead of her being the expert and me being the patient, us being co-communicators about my body. That's what I'd like to see ...'

Sharing information

Sharing information with the client about the initial examination and about every component of treatment also helps the client to develop a sense of safety. Information must flow both from the

---

Box 7.1 Principles of sensitive practice that facilitate survivors' feelings of safety

- Respect
- Rapport
- Sharing control
- Sharing information
- Respecting boundaries
- Fostering a mutual learning process
- Consideration of the ebbs and flows of living with past abuse
- Demonstrating an awareness of prevalence of violence and child sexual abuse

clinician to the client and from the client to the clinician. The onus for developing and maintaining this two-way flow of information rests with the clinician: she or he should explain the examination and treatment and seek ongoing feedback about reactions to treatment and about the client's perception of progress:

'I found quite often, when you go to a doctor or physiotherapist, they automatically assume that you have some kind of knowledge of their job outline … And why should I know? I didn't go to school for that, so it's really frustrating. And they expect you to know something about it …'

Respect for boundaries

We believed that 'respect for boundaries' merited recognition as a fundamental principle even though it is also manifested in other principles of sensitive practice. Through respect for the client and the sharing of information and control, the health professional can demonstrate a genuine effort to be sensitive to boundaries. The clinician must consider the power imbalance between professionals and clients in all efforts to respect physical, psychological and emotional boundaries. By demonstrating respect for and sensitivity to boundaries, the clinician may also serve as a model for the survivor who is learning to establish healthy boundaries in her life.

Fostering a mutual learning process

The principles outlined above may reflect experiences that the survivor did not have as a child and is therefore learning for the first time as an adult. She may need encouragement in her journey to become a full, active participant in her own health care. The following woman's words remind us that learning to be an active participant means more than just following a health professional's advice:

'That assertiveness of [saying] "no" takes a long time to get … it was somebody else giving me permission that allowed me to say "no" until I could learn to give myself permission [to do so] …'

At the same time, the clinician is learning about working with survivors. The learning process is not easy and participants pointed out that errors will be made. They went on to suggest that

to address such mistakes, the clinician needs to acknowledge his or her mistake, offer an apology and subsequently discuss the uncomfortable situation with the client to resolve the problems that may have arisen.

Consideration of ebbs and flows

Neither coping with the effects nor healing from child sexual abuse is a linear process. As a result, the survivor may vary in the degree to which she is able to tolerate and participate in treatment at various times. Fluctuations in the survivor's level of tolerance may occur rapidly (from day to day, for example) or may develop over longer periods of time. To address the possibility for such changes, the clinician must repeatedly 'check in' with the client and be willing to adjust the treatment approach accordingly:

'If I say today, "No. I don't think I can handle you doing that", not to be treated like some sort of baby … or … "What's your problem?" kind of thing … but to accept that when I say, "No. You can't touch my neck today. You know, maybe tomorrow – but you can't touch it today …".'

Demonstrating an awareness of the prevalence and sequelae of violence and child sexual abuse

Many survivors look for indicators of the clinician's awareness of issues of violence, trauma and abuse. Such demonstrations range from external indicators such as posters and pamphlets from a local sexual assault centre, to incorporating the principles and guidelines for sensitive practice into the clinician's everyday interactions with the client:

'… I'm way more interested in … how much awareness [the health professional has] around trauma. So, that holds a lot of weight with me.'

Guidelines for sensitive practice

In addition to the principles of sensitive practice, we have developed guidelines that address specific components of clinical practice from the initial examination to discharge, which the reader will find presented in the handbook. Within the context of guidelines for sensitive practice, the issue of disclosure requires particular attention. Is knowledge of a client's history of abuse relevant to physical therapy treatment? Most survivors felt that the abuse they had experienced as children affected their health and health care. They described a number of ways that this could be manifested. It may be seen primarily in the survivor's need to feel safe, to be respected and feel in control. It may also be that the survivor is apprehensive of or has encountered 'triggers', which resulted in flashbacks or sudden strong emotions related to past abuse, during previous interactions with health professionals. The survivor may be seeking treatment for a chronic condition that stemmed from injuries sustained as a child or for pain that she suspects is being aggravated by past abuse.

We have described two independent, although related, forms of disclosure. The first is initiated by the clinician through task-centred inquiry. The clinician should inquire about the task-centred sensitivities and discomforts during the initial examination. Through such inquiry, the client can share specific information that is immediately pertinent to the treatment without revealing other personal information she is not prepared to share. The clinician can make such enquiries using both direct questions (e.g. 'Are you sensitive to having someone touch your legs? Knees? Feet?') and open-ended questions (e.g. 'Is there anything else you feel I should know before we begin the examination?'). The information that the survivor discloses (such as problems tolerating touch or certain body positions) can be addressed as the examination and treatment proceed. The clinician needs to employ task-specific enquiries to address sensitivities and difficulties on an ongoing basis, for example when body language or poor treatment adherence suggests unexpressed discomfort or problems, and as treatment changes.

The second form of disclosure is disclosure of past abuse. Regardless of whether health professionals asked about past abuse or not, survivors told us that they decided about whether to disclose based primarily on whether they felt safe enough, whether the clinician was trustworthy, and how they thought the clinician would react to the disclosure. As one woman put it: 'Some people go "ahhh" and other people go "uhhh".' Participant opinions on whether the clinician should ask about past abuse ranged from 'never' to 'yes with every new client'. Thus, an inquiry about past abuse will be welcomed by some clients and experienced very negatively by others.

WHY THE CHOSEN RESEARCH METHOD FITS THE RESEARCH PURPOSE

Two considerations guided the logic of the research design and methodology used in this study: (1) relevance and (2) the power differentials between clients and professionals.

Relevance

'We define action research as research in which the validity and value of research results are tested through collaborative insider–professional researcher knowledge generation and application processes in projects of social change that aim to increase fairness, wellness, and self-determination' (Greenwood & Levin 2000, p. 94).

Using the literature about child sexual abuse survivors, and our own knowledge, we could have taken a more 'scientific' approach to this study. For example, we could have developed a list of issues that should presumably occupy the mind of survivors when being treated by physical therapists (e.g. removal of clothing, touch, etc.). We could have then developed a questionnaire related to these issues and conducted a survey to identify those most frequently endorsed. While this approach would have facilitated a larger sample than the design we used, it would also have generated less meaningful data. For example, knowing that a large proportion of survivors were concerned with being touched was less relevant for our purpose than knowing what makes this touch a troubling experience or what makes it a positive healing experience. Similarly, we could have presented survivors with a list of physical therapy practices and asked them to rank these practices in terms of sensitivity to their needs.

This would have produced a neatly ranked list of sensitive practices; however, this ranking would have been less useful, because it would exclude the powerful experiences of survivors that assert the need for clinicians to reflect on ways of relating to clients and continually explore practices that are sensitive to clients' needs.

To be relevant, we believed that it was necessary to capture the experiential knowledge of both survivors and health professionals on their own terms, without the constraints and guidance of a predefined framework. Given the lack of previous research in this area, it was also important that the ideas emerging from our study originate with the people most knowledgeable about the subject matter. Thus, we needed a research design that would facilitate the exchange of knowledge between two groups of experts: child sexual abuse survivors and physical therapists.

The grounded theory approach (Glaser & Strauss 1967), with its focus on the emergence of theory from data, was clearly the most suitable for the first phase of the study. The interviews with women survivors began with a general 'grand tour' question (Spradley 1979), which allowed these participants to take us through their experiences by highlighting the sites of their choice rather than those chosen by us. Although grounded theory has been influenced by positivism, the adoption of this approach does not require a positivist stance (Charmaz 2000) and can be used, as in this study, to understand subjective realities. Nevertheless, the rigorous and systematic analyses required for the development of a grounded theory may be an advantage in the health field, which is dominated by positivist thinking. Thus, this approach facilitated both the collection of relevant data and its acceptance by health professionals.

While the data collected in the first phase reflected the subjective experiences of child sexual abuse survivors, the second and third phases were designed to use this information for the generation of usable knowledge. The data from the interviews were sufficiently rich to permit the drawing of our own conclusions for the development of practices that are sensitive to the needs of women survivors of child sexual abuse. However, in order to be relevant, these ideas had to be derived through 'dialoguing with a polyphony of voices' (Flyvbjerg 2001). In this process, the researchers do not claim final authority, but develop knowledge through input to the ongoing dialogue and praxis.

Flyvbjerg (2001) reminds us that 'the development of social research is inhibited by the fact that researchers tend to work with problems in which the answer to the question "If you are wrong about this, who will notice?" is "Nobody"' (p. 132). He suggests that this problem of relevance can be addressed by anchoring the research in the context studied and by getting 'close to the phenomenon or group whom one studies during data collection, and remain close during the phases of data analysis, feedback and publication of results' (p. 132). The dialogue we facilitated in the second phase brought together representatives of the groups who would have noticed and cared if the knowledge produced through this research was wrong or impractical. The survivors in these groups had an interest in this dialogue because the guidelines they were developing were intended to improve the quality of health care provided to them and to other survivors. The physical therapists in these groups had an interest in making these guidelines workable for themselves and their colleagues. The integration of their perspectives was essential for creating a balance between the ideal and the manageable. In the final stages of the study, we expanded the 'hermeneutic fusion of horizons' (Flyvbjerg 2001, p. 132) to include the views of other survivors and professionals through written and verbal feedback on drafts of the *Handbook on Sensitive Practice*.

Power

No discourse is unequivocally oppressive or always emancipatory. The researcher's methodology must take account of the complex and unstable process according to which discourses can be both an instrument of power and its effect, but also an obstacle, a point of resistance or a starting point for a counterposing strategy. Discourses thus transfer and produce power (Flyvbjerg 2001, p. 124).

While the design of this study enhanced its relevance by facilitating the delivery of the original voices of survivors to professionals in terms that were acceptable to both groups, it also took into consideration the power differentials between the two groups.

While participatory action research addresses the power differentials between researchers and the people they study, it does not necessarily consider the inequalities among research participants. Although our study included elements of action research design, we did not begin with the definition of objectives and questions through a collaborative process. Instead, we initiated this study based on the assumption that knowledge related to the relationship between physical therapists and survivors can improve the quality of care provided by professionals. The use of a grounded theory exploration of the experiences of child sexual abuse survivors as our starting point was designed to address the imbalance between the expertise accorded to clients and that of professionals.

This approach allowed survivors the opportunity to express themselves without the constraints of practicality. Thus, we avoided the common context for communication between clients and health professionals that tends to be dominated by considerations of what the latter can or cannot do. Although these considerations were central to the dialogue in the second phase of the study, survivors entered this dialogue equipped with their own knowledge and experiences, and empowered by the wisdom of other survivors. In other words, they had a theory about their needs as a counterbalance to the theory that guided the professionals who participated in these groups.

The importance of equipping survivors with their own theory cannot be overemphasized in the context of evidence-based practice. Unlike health professionals, survivors – and for that matter most client populations – do not have an institutionalized group identity with a body of knowledge to help construct this identity. Thus, clients are not considered 'expert witnesses', and the evidence they provide to inform our practice can be easily disregarded as impressionistic, idiosyncratic and subjective. If qualitative research is indeed about 'the generation of communicative process' and its aim is 'the establishment of productive forms of relationship' (Gergen & Gergen 2000), we cannot

ignore the power differentials between the participant groups engaged in our studies.

HOW OUR FINDINGS COULD BE USED TO CRITIQUE AND DEVELOP PRACTICE

A number of the principles and guidelines of sensitive practice are also embedded within models of client-centred care (e.g. College of Physiotherapists of Ontario 2001, Law et al 1995, Stewart et al 1995). Sensitive practice can, however, be seen as a way to 'fine tune' components of client-centred care because it encourages clinicians to move beyond the general goals of client-centred practice in its recognition of the prevalence of abuse and knowledge that factors related to abuse can dominate many survivors' needs during treatment. Survivors repeatedly emphasized that without ongoing attention to the survivor's need to feel safe, to be respected and feel in control, they experienced difficulties that could adversely affect their health and health care, and may actually prohibit them from continuing treatment. This underscores the importance of clinicians' efforts to regard sensitive practice as a necessary refinement or addition to the elements of patient-centred care.

This research provides a number of challenges to practitioners. Two such challenges relate to the breadth of our understanding of the client and the extent of our attempts to practise holistically. Client-centred care emphasizes the need to understand the whole person: the disease, the illness (that is, the ways that the client experiences the disease), the person (including the stage in the life cycle and family of origin) and the context (including family system, culture, work, etc.) (Weston & Brown 1995, p. 166). Our interviews with survivors support the psychological literature in illustrating ways in which past abuse has affected all of these elements of survivors' lives. These findings support the physical therapists' re-examination of the breadth of their interactions with clients. In the third phase of our study, for example, many clinician and students indicated that they were more comfortable with not knowing that a client had a history of abuse. Some clinicians and students did not see it as directly relevant to their work with clients. Many felt ill prepared to deal with such information if disclosed to them. If physical therapists are to practise holistically, how can we reconcile these perspectives with developing a comprehensive understanding of the client?

Applying the principles and guidelines of sensitive practice to all clients – in the same way that we use 'universal precautions' to prevent infection – can assist in addressing this dilemma. Sensitive practice represents actions that survivors have told us facilitate feeling safe during treatment. Feeling safe means that the client perceives she is working and connecting with a trustworthy clinician. This, in turn, may allow her to explore her health in a broader way. Thus, regardless of whether the client has disclosed, using sensitive practice is likely to help the clinician to get to know and understand the whole person. We believe that all health professionals should incorporate sensitive practice as part of their client-centred approach to practice. It follows that, during the training of physical therapists, instructors should include sensitive practice not only in theory and clinical examples but also by modelling of the behaviours in their interactions with students.

This research provides a challenge for clinicians to revisit their ideas about whether they could employ additional techniques to enhance holistic practice. Clinicians in phase three spoke about working with clients whose presenting problems appeared to be linked to their mental health (just as survivors described the interconnectedness of their physical and mental health). We see this borne out in a growing body of evidence that demonstrates the physiological links between mind and body (e.g. Heim et al 2000, van der Kolk 1996). This evidence speaks to the wisdom of clinician and client joining together to create new healthcare teams composed of the client and the various health practitioners with whom she works. Perhaps by working together in non-traditional ways, a team can bridge the gap that the current dualistic perspective on health creates and thereby demonstrate a more client-centred holistic notion of function, care, context and healing (McWhinney 1995, p. 14).

The principles and guidelines of sensitive practice may at first overwhelm the clinician who has limited time for each client. Nevertheless, clinicians may want to reflect on the possibility that resources, time and energy are wasted when treatment is delivered in a way that is not acceptable to or usable by clients. We need to recognize that past abuse can intrude on treatment, affecting such things as client adherence to treatment regimens, attendance or action the client can take to prevent a recurrence of the condition. The cost related to non-adherence to treatment and the lost opportunity to share information about the condition, the body, the importance of self-care and other forms of health promotion and disease prevention should not be underestimated. The amount of time saved by not actively relating to the 'non-somatic' needs of clients may be an illusion.

Both our research process and product (Schachter et al 2001) demonstrate how qualitative research can contribute to the evidence base for clinical practice. The research process shows how clients can inform us about their lives, help us understand how our actions affect them, and how we can work in ways that can help them benefit from clinical interventions. The process we used can be applied by clinicians in a number of ways. On an individual level, this process reflects the use of client-centred care. The clinician could also use the process by conducting focus groups with individuals with a particular condition to gain further understanding about how the condition and care of the condition are experienced by individuals. On a larger scale, practitioners can form partnerships with researchers to carry out the whole process that brings the realities of clients and clinicians together. The rich data and practical knowledge that emerge from this process reinforce a client-centred orientation to the generation of evidence-based clinical practice.

REFERENCES

Charmaz K 2000 Grounded theory: objectivists and constructivist methods. In: Denzin NK, Lincoln YS (eds) Handbook of qualitative research. 2nd edn. Sage, Thousand Oaks, CA; pp. 509–538

College of Physiotherapists of Ontario 2001 Are you providing patient centred care? College of Physiotherapists of Ontario, Toronto

Felitti VJ 1991 Long-term medical consequences of incest, rape, and molestation. Southern Medical Journal 84:328–331

Finestone HM, Stenn P, Davies F et al 2000 Chronic pain and health care utilization in women with a history of childhood sexual abuse. Child Abuse and Neglect 24:547–556

Finkelhor D 1994 Current information on the scope and nature of child sexual abuse. The Future of Children 4:31–53

Flyvbjerg B 2001 Making social science matter. Cambridge University Press, Cambridge

Fry R 1993 Invited review: adult physical illness and childhood sexual abuse. Journal of Psychosomatic Research 37:89–103

Gergen MM, Gergen KJ 2000 Qualitative inquiry: tensions and transformations. In: Denzin NK, Lincoln YS (eds) Handbook of qualitative research. 2nd edn. Sage, Thousand Oaks, CA; pp. 1025–1046

Glaser BG, Strauss AL 1967 The discovery of grounded theory. Aldine, Chicago

Greenwood DJ, Levin M 2000 Reconstructing the relationships between universities and society through action research. In: Denzin NK, Lincoln YS (eds) Handbook of qualitative research. 2nd edn. Sage, Thousand Oaks, CA; pp. 85–106

Harrop-Griffeths J, Katon W, Walker E et al 1988 The association between chronic pelvic pain, psychiatric diagnoses and childhood sexual abuse. Obstetrics and Gynecology 71:589–594

Heim C, Newport J, Heit S et al 2000 Pituitary–adrenal and autonomic responses to stress in women after sexual and physical abuse in childhood. Journal of the American Medical Association 284:592–597

Law M, Baptiste S, Mills J 1995 Client-centred practice: what does it mean and does it make a difference? Canadian Journal of Occupational Therapy 62(5):250–257

Laws A 1993 Does a history of sexual abuse in childhood play a role in women's medical problems? A review. Journal of Women's Health 2:165–172

Lechner ME, Vogel ME, Garcia-Shelton LM et al 1993 Self-reported medical problems of adult female survivors of childhood sexual abuse. Journal of Family Practice 36:633–638

McWhinney IR 1995 Why we need a new clinical method. In: Stewart M, Brown, JB, Weston WW et al (eds) Patient-centred medicine. Transforming the clinical method. Sage, Thousand Oaks, CA; pp. 1–18

Reason P 1988 The co-operative inquiry group. In: Reason P (ed) Human inquiry in action: developments in new paradigm research. Sage, London; pp. 18–39

Reason P 1994 Three approaches to participative inquiry. In: Denzin NK, Lincoln YS (eds) Handbook of qualitative research. Sage, Thousand Oaks, CA; pp. 324–339

Reiter RC, Gambone JC 1990 Demographic and historic variables in women with idiopathic chronic pelvic pain. Obstetrics and Gynecology 75:428–432

Schachter CL, Stalker CA, Teram E 2001 Handbook on sensitive practice for health professionals – lessons from women survivors of childhood sexual abuse. National Clearinghouse on Family Violence, Family Violence Prevention Unit, Centre for Healthy Human Development, Health Canada, Ottawa (http://www.hc-sc.gc.ca/nc-cn). Online. Available: http://www.hc-sc.gc.ca/hppb/familyviolence/pdfs/handbook%20e.pdf 18 March 2003

Spradley JP 1979 The ethnographic interview. Holt Rinehart & Winston, New York

Springs FE, Friedrich W 1992 Health risk behaviors and medical sequela of childhood sexual abuse. Mayo Clinic Proceedings 67:527–532

Stewart M, Brown JB, Weston WW et al 1995 Patient-centred medicine. Transforming the clinical method. Sage, Thousand Oaks, CA

van der Kolk BA 1996 The body keeps the score: approaches to the psychobiology of posttraumatic stress disorder. In: van der Kolk BA, McFarlane AC, Weisaith L (eds) Traumatic stress. The effects of overwhelming experiences on mind, body, and society. Guilford Press, New York; pp. 214–241

Walker EA, Katon WJ, Roy-Byrne PP et al 1993 Histories of sexual victimization in patients with irritable bowel syndrome or inflammatory bowel disease. American Journal of Psychiatry 150:502–506

Weston WW, Brown JB 1995 Teaching the patient-centred method: practical tips. In: Stewart M, Brown JB, Weston WW et al (eds) Patient-centred medicine. Transforming the clinical method. Sage, Thousand Oaks, CA; pp. 159–182

FURTHER READING

Schachter CL, Stalker CA, Teram E 2001 Handbook on sensitive practice for health professionals: lessons from women survivors of childhood sexual abuse. National Clearinghouse on Family Violence, Family Violence Prevention Unit, Centre for Healthy Human Development, Health Canada, Ottawa (http://www.hc-sc.gc.ca/nc-cn). Online. Available: http://www.hc-sc.gc.ca/hppb/familyviolence/pdfs/handbook%20e.pdf 18 March 2003

Stalker CA, Schachter CL, Teram E 1999 Facilitating effective relationships between survivors of childhood sexual abuse and health care professionals. Affilia: Journal of Women and Social Work 14(2):176–198

Teram E, Schachter CL, Stalker CA 1999 Opening the doors to disclosure: childhood sexual abuse survivors reflect on telling physical therapists about their trauma. Physiotherapy 85(2):88–97

8

How qualitative research evidence can inform and challenge occupational therapy practice

Karen Rebeiro

OVERVIEW

This chapter is an exemplar of evidence-based practice and service delivery. Through a series of qualitative studies, Karen Rebeiro and her co-researchers (mental health consumers) explored the unmet needs of mental health consumers, developed a collaborative, occupation-based mental health programme, and evaluated this initiative on an ongoing basis. The initial research had been concerned with addressing the question: 'If occupational therapy practice in mental health is defined by the use of or application of occupation, what is the evidence to support this practice?' Evidence from this study led to further studies such that not solely occupational therapy theory but modes of practice and models of service delivery became firmly grounded in a credible and relevant evidence base.

K.H.

INTRODUCTION

This chapter describes a series of research studies that led to the development of a collaborative, occupation-based mental health initiative known as the Northern Initiative for Social Action (NISA). What began as a clinical irritation concerning both the use of occupation-as-therapy and the paucity of evidence to support occupational therapy practice in mental health dovetailed into a series of studies that challenged traditional modes of service delivery for this client group and that led to changes in both professional practice and service provision. Specifically, this chapter addresses the following:

- What prompted the research?
- Why qualitative methods?
- What evidence was discovered by qualitative research that subsequently informed the author's clinical practice?
- How was the evidence applied in clinical practice?
- How has the evidence challenged current ways of practising occupational therapy?

WHAT PROMPTED THE RESEARCH?

The series of research projects that inform this chapter were triggered by a deep-seated frustration with clinical practice. Specifically, I was frustrated by continual requests to explain what I did as an occupational therapist and to define a practice with which I was increasingly uncomfortable and uncertain. Despite my good intentions (Townsend 1998), and despite what I considered to be a fairly successful clinical practice in mental health, I became increasingly uncomfortable with my own practice, with my profession, with my own perceived inability to make a difference for people and, specifically, with my limited power to effect greater change within a system that I perceived to be ineffective for clients.

The following comprises the issues and questions that have prompted my research in graduate school and since then:

1. What is occupational therapy about? What is our role?
2. What is it that occupational therapists do that makes the profession unique within the healthcare system and of value to the public?
3. What is the evidence that supports these roles and functions in health care?

I knew at a basic level that occupational therapists were concerned with occupation. However, I recognized that this was neither explicit nor clearly evident in my practice or that of my colleagues. A brief review of the literature could readily demonstrate that a clear parameter of occupational therapy practice did not exist. My experience as an occupational therapist suggested that our professional tendency was to do what we deemed to be in the best interests of the client, and to fill in gaps in service. Clearly, filling in perceived gaps in the delivery of services would do little to explain our *raison d'être* to clients, the profession or the public. I also knew from experience that my value to the system had a great deal to do with my own clinical skills and relationships with clients, and perhaps less to do with my education or training as an occupational therapist. Although I attempted to utilize 'occupation' in my practice and to 'enable the occupational performance' of my clients, my practice was largely structured to promote verbal therapy and a quick turnaround of clients, and this appeared to be based more upon economics and less upon being 'client centred'.

Experience had taught me that the system did – and does not – necessarily foster a continuum of care for clients. Often the clients would become lost in the mental health system, which appeared to work well for the professionals but less well for the clients it was ostensibly created to help. There remained a gap between the two systems – hospital and community. The system appeared to be tailored to work for those individuals who held the decision-making power in my organization. The organization of mental health systems and the influence of power and decision-making is a phenomenon that has been described extensively by Elizabeth Townsend (1998) in her book, *Good Intentions Overruled*. In her ethnography of the organization of mental health systems in Eastern Canada, Townsend (1998) describes how systems often render occupational therapists powerless to realize their good intentions and the work they aim to do. Further, Townsend highlights how, in the absence of significant systemic changes, the structure of mental health organizations will continue to thwart any good intentions of occupational therapists whose aim is to enable the occupational performance of their clients. Townsend's research has made an incredible difference to my understanding of the system in which I work. Her ethnography helped me to understand the importance of research, and of building an evidence base to inform and effect real change.

WHY QUALITATIVE METHODS?

In graduate school I learned about a variety of research methods that could potentially help me to find some of the answers to my many questions. I learned about traditional quantitative methods of conducting research, but these methods seemed neither to fit nor to be appropriate to the questions for which I sought answers. I needed methods that would allow for, or facilitate, an exploratory approach to the research, and be open-ended enough to facilitate client input and participation in the process (Cook 2001). Qualitative methods seemed a natural fit, and appeared well suited to the phenomenon under investigation, namely, mental health consumers' experiences of the system, of engaging in occupation, and of their ability to seek out and secure meaningful occupational opportunities in their community. I especially liked how qualitative researchers recognized that clients were the ones with the knowledge of their experiences, the authors of their own stories. I appreciated the open-ended nature of the questioning that allowed the client or participant to lead the research process. Qualitative methods, for me, seemed congruent with client centredness.

The qualitative methods that I have employed have included the long or active interview (Holstein & Gubrium 1995, McCracken 1988), participant observation (Jorgenson 1989), participatory action research (Whyte 1991) and the use of focus groups (Morgan 1988). As a general rule, I attempt to incorporate multiple methods into my research, as these are appropriate to inform the research process and enhance the trustworthiness of any findings (Lincoln & Guba 1985).

THE RESEARCH IMPERATIVE

The first task after identifying a question is to go to the literature. The question that guided my review of the literature was: 'If occupational therapy practice in mental health is defined by the use of or application of occupation, what is the evidence to support this practice?'

Unfortunately, an extensive review of the occupational therapy literature did not yield any studies that supported the use of occupation in occupational therapy mental health practice (Rebeiro 1998). There were many discussion papers about the use of occupation or activity in psychosocial occupational therapy practice, but I could not find a single study that researched the benefits of using occupation as the basis of practice or that targeted occupational engagement or performance as the outcome or dependent variable of practice (Rebeiro 1998). It was evident that occupational therapists were slow to engage in research that either defined or supported practice. Clearly, unless occupational therapists become serious about conducting research that will enable us to define and justify our practice, we are at serious risk of losing our place in the current healthcare arena, which increasingly demands an evidence base to inform and support practice (Rebeiro 1998, Townsend & Rebeiro 2001).

SEEKING QUALITATIVE EVIDENCE TO INFORM PRACTICE

The following evidence is derived from individual research projects, each of which taught me something about occupational therapy practice and theory. What follows is a brief, chronological synopsis of the evidence uncovered or discovered by a series of research studies that dovetailed, one into another, and that became driven by the many questions that remained to be answered at the conclusion of the previous research study. This process is illustrated in Figure 8.1.

STUDY ONE: THE WOMEN'S GROUP

For my Master's thesis, I had the opportunity to study a group of women with serious, persistent mental illnesses who met on a weekly basis in an occupation-based support group that I had started in 1991. Prior to the formation of this group, these women had been readmitted to hospital on a regular basis and I had initially believed that if they had an opportunity for support on a weekly basis, in addition to the opportunity to work collaboratively on a group project, this might help them to do better. At the time of the study, approximately 5 years after starting the group, none of these women had been readmitted to hospital. Occupation was the sole factor that differentiated membership in this group from the other services and programmes previously available to them, which led to my hunch that their success at staying out of the hospital

might have something to do with their engagement in occupation. However, I did not have research evidence to support this premise. I decided to investigate their experience of participation in the group by asking the question, 'What is the experience of occupational engagement for members of the women's group?', in an effort to understand the meaning and purpose of occupation for this group, in addition to learning what factors contributed to group members staying out of hospital.

The women's group study was my introduction into the world of research. It was a group that I was familiar with, but with whom I had not had direct contact for over 2 years. The study utilized several methods, including in-depth interviews and participant observation as a group member for a period of 25 weeks – 16 weeks as an observer and 9 weeks as a group participant. I certainly would not have learned as much about the women's experiences had I limited my methods to in-depth interviewing. The insights that I gained from being a participant in the group cannot be emphasized enough. In combination, the two methods provided me with credible and trustworthy findings upon which to inform my practice.

The evidence uncovered

The findings of this study are articulated in more depth elsewhere (Rebeiro 1997, 2001a,b, Rebeiro & Cook 1999). Briefly, the evidence uncovered which subsequently informed practice comprised the following themes.

Occupation: opportunity, not prescription

It was evident that only the clients/participants could decide what held personal meaning, interest and purpose for them with respect to the occupations in which they engaged (Rebeiro 2000). Traditionally, occupational therapists have done a disservice to clients, under the guise of 'professionalism'. Perceiving themselves to be 'experts', they decided what the clients' needs were, what their priorities should be in therapy, what occupations were provided as therapy,

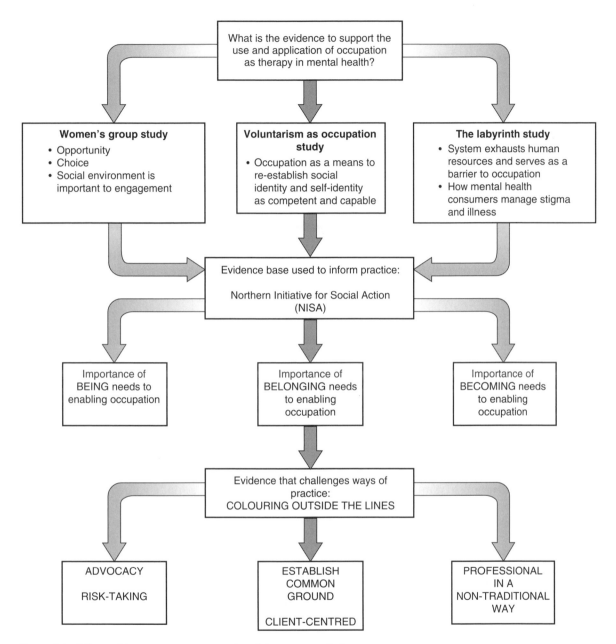

Figure 8.1   What evidence supports occupational therapy practice?

and what ought to be meaningful for the client. Rather than collaboratively choosing an occupational path, therapists allowed the economics or time constraints of practice to determine which occupations could be provided for clients. The women's experiences clearly demonstrated that occupational therapists need to foster client choice and participation in occupations that have value or personal meaning for the client both in hospital and in their lives beyond the hospital. As one of the participants in the women's group told me when speaking about doing a tile trivet: 'What do they think we are, morons?' Another participant stated: 'anybody knows that a choice of three [things] is no choice at all when clearly there are millions of choices of things to do in this world'.

Importance of the social environment

During the in-depth interviews, the women kept emphasizing how important the members of the group were to them, but I was not tuned into what they were trying to tell me, because I was intent on learning about occupation and the experience of occupational engagement. It became clear to me only upon becoming a group participant, and both watching and participating in the dynamics of the group, that the social environment and support in the group (what I termed 'affirmation') was critical in bolstering individuals' courage to engage in occupations or to experiment with the trial-and-error aspects of new learning. Despite successful completion of a variety of occupational projects, the women did not gain a sense of themselves as competent persons unless their participation in and/or completion of their occupational project was confirmed by the other group members (what I termed 'confirmation'). It became a sort of feedback loop between the occupation and the social environment of the group. The reciprocity between members and their occupations assisted the participants to gain a sense of themselves not only as worthwhile and valuable human beings – rather than as mental health clients – but also as competent individuals. This renewed perception of themselves and of their abilities contributed to 'looking forward' to other groups, gatherings and events in their lives. They anticipated further involvement in the group in order to continue feeling good – a stage I termed 'anticipation'. Members would then actively seek out, explore and participate in further and different occupations both within the group and beyond, a process I coined 'occupational spin-off' (Rebeiro 1997, 2001a, Rebeiro & Cook 1999). Spin-off was evident when the members were actively participating in occupations beyond the group and within the community, and this was largely driven by members' desire to continue feeling good.

Despite learning some fairly important insights about the experience of engaging in occupations and its importance to members' sense of self and mental health, the women suggested that the reason they remained in this hospital-based group was because they did not perceive that similar opportunities or supportive environments existed in their community. It was this revelation that prompted me to undertake another study to explore what in fact consumers did on a daily basis within their community and what opportunities they had for meaningful occupation.

STUDY TWO: VOLUNTARISM AS OCCUPATION

In seeking to understand further the experience of engaging in meaningful occupation for mental health consumers, a single-case study design was employed to explore and then describe the personal experience of voluntarism for one individual with schizophrenia (Rebeiro & Allen 1998). Non-participant observation and a series of in-depth interviews were used to collect the data. The findings supported occupational therapy's theoretical literature in that the individual perceived his volunteer position to be both a meaningful and a purposeful occupation. John's voluntary work was perceived to be a socially valued occupation that provided him with a means to achieve a social identity as a contributing member of the community. Further, volunteering was identified as a means to re-establish a sense of self as being competent instead of being a mental health patient.

This study also highlighted for occupational therapists the influence of stigma on active and meaningful participation in occupation. John spoke candidly about having to conceal his illness identity in order to be respected and judged on his work performance rather than upon preconceived notions about mental illness or schizophrenia. His insights are mirrored in the consumer literature (Deegan 1992, Estroff 1989, Leete 1989) and shed light on the need for professionals to provide safe and accepting environments (Davidson et al 2001), rather than relegating mental health clients to the margins of society (Goffman 1963).

STUDY THREE: THE LABYRINTH OF COMMUNITY MENTAL HEALTH

The third in the series of research studies focused on the experience of seeking, finding and participating in personally meaningful occupation within the community (Rebeiro 1999). The following section outlines what I learned in this research project.

The methods employed in this study were participant observation or field research for a period of 18 months, in-depth interviews, a survey of community mental health programmes and document reviews. The 'labyrinth' study was my opportunity to meet and converse with several mental health consumers who were residing in the community and who were therefore in their own space. I was able to ask them directly about what they did on a daily basis with their time and what opportunities they perceived to exist for them to participate in personally meaningful and socially valued occupations. From their experiences I learned a great deal about how the mental health 'system' was exhausting consumers and maintaining people in a position of dependency. The labyrinth of community mental health systems and services had far-reaching implications for consumers' participation in occupation.

The evidence uncovered

The labyrinth study was an important research project through which I learned that many of the processes, systems and ways of practice in mental health services were perceived to be a deterrent to consumers seeking, finding, obtaining and maintaining involvement in occupation within the community. Four primary issues were identified through data analysis.

Barriers to participation in meaningful occupation within communities

One of the major findings of the labyrinth study was how mental health systems that govern community mental healthcare practice actually serve as deterrents or barriers to mental health consumers' pursuit of and participation in occupation. In general, the arduous rules and regulations imposed at the municipal, provincial and federal levels of government tend to serve as disincentives to consumers of mental health services who might otherwise consider return to work as a viable option. Instead, they are told that if they are able to volunteer, then they must be able to work; if they can work part-time, then they must be able to work full-time; if they are able to work full-time, then they do not need disability or social support. The ongoing and prevalent threat to basic financial support was a primary reason cited by consumers for their lack of involvement in occupation (paid or voluntary) within the community. Despite their recognition that they could be doing more, or their desire to do something meaningful with their time and their lives, many consumers were afraid to risk losing the support they needed to pay for their rent, basic needs and the high costs of the medications they had to take to control symptoms of the illness. Eventually, consumers come to a point of being so frustrated with the mental health and income support systems that they lose hope for anything better and become acclimatized to living a life that does not include work – or any form of meaningful occupation. Despite governments' declared intent to foster the recovery of mental health consumers, existing policies and funding formulas appear to prohibit mental health consumers from becoming full and contributing citizens within our communities.

Importance of simplifying the maze of referral, access and participation

A second finding concerns the labyrinth of referral processes that consumers need to navigate to enlist the support of the system. Consumers did not perceive that the system was accessible, nor did they perceive that the system was geared to assisting consumers eventually to exit the system or to have a life beyond the confines of the mental health system. Higgins (2001) noted that, while much discussion centres on how to make the system more accessible, nobody talks about how to get out of the system.

The referral process in the mental health system was also identified as being problematic to consumers who sought involvement in occupation. First, they did not perceive that those mental health professionals with whom they were involved either encouraged their involvement in occupation or considered this to be a priority. This finding was confirmed by the survey of mental health agencies, which identified that few resources (human or fiscal) were dedicated to assisting mental health consumers become involved in occupation. Consumers did not perceive that they had choices within the system or the opportunity to negotiate a return to work or more active involvement within their community.

The impact of stigma on community participation

Stigma was also seen to be a major barrier to mental health consumers' movement beyond traditional services and to their pursuit of and participation in meaningful occupation. Stigma was felt to be related both to the side-effects of the medications consumers took to control their symptoms, especially the powerful antipsychotic medications, and to the effects of being a mental health consumer and in receipt of a disability pension. Many commented on the stigma related to being in a position of financial dependency, which essentially means poverty. Folks perceived that the limited funds they received as a result of their disability barely provided for the basic needs in life, such as housing and food, let alone for transportation costs, clothing, haircuts, etc., to remove the stigma relating to looking poor or 'like a mental health client'. Therapists need to be aware of the energy expense incurred in managing illness identity and how this subsequently affects occupational choices and performance.

Negotiating the labyrinth: a full-time occupation

The variety and extent of referrals that required management by the mental health consumer were perceived to exhaust their resources. These included visits with their psychiatrist, meetings with case management workers or their disability support person, and managing medications and their side-effects. Many participants stated that chasing referrals and figuring out the labyrinth of

services that were in place to assist them constituted their daily existence. Further, this process exhausted their mental and physical energy to such a degree that they did not perceive themselves to have any energy left for their pursuit of and participation in occupation. Fulfilling their role as a mental health consumer within an inflexible system was becoming a full-time occupation that engaged a great deal of their lives. Many people did not perceive a way out or have hope for anything better.

SUMMARY OF FINDINGS FROM THE THREE STUDIES

- The importance of generating an evidence base to support and define occupational therapy practice in mental health
- The importance of the environment to enabling engagement in occupation
- The importance of hopefulness
- The importance of providing opportunity, rather than prescription of occupation
- The phenomenon of successful occupational performance spinning off to other occupational engagement beyond the group and into the community
- The importance of volunteering to re-establishing a sense of self as competent and capable
- The importance of volunteering to re-establishing a social identity in the community
- The importance of volunteering as a means to community involvement and to seeking other occupational opportunities
- The labyrinth or maze of programmes and services that get in the way of mental health consumers finding and securing participation in meaningful occupation within their community
- The importance of simplifying the system of referral, access and participation
- How the labyrinth of mental health programmes and services becomes a full-time occupation for many mental health consumers, essentially depleting a great deal of their energy and leaving little for the

pursuit or participation in meaningful occupation

- How social stigma affects one's confidence to explore and participate fully in the community
- How managing stigma and illness identity serves to distance consumers from their community
- The importance of reducing or eliminating power differentials or hierarchies in providing services
- The importance of 'real work' versus 'make work' opportunities.

Unfortunately, many of the systemic barriers identified in the labyrinth study are currently beyond the scope and practice of most occupational therapists. However, that does not negate the need to appreciate the issues and barriers that many mental health consumers face daily within their communities, nor eliminate professional responsibility to address these barriers in practice. Many opportunities exist for occupational therapists to advocate for and participate in fostering real occupational opportunities for mental health consumers within communities, so that they may have hope and a chance to move beyond the system.

APPLICATION OF THE EVIDENCE TO SERVICE DELIVERY: NORTHERN INITIATIVE FOR SOCIAL ACTION

The information learned from these research studies has been applied to a theoretical model of practice known as occupational spin-off (Rebeiro 1997, 2001a, Rebeiro & Cook 1999), which has been further refined and applied to a clinical model, known as NISA (Rebeiro et al 2001). NISA – the Northern Initiative for Social Action – evolved directly from evidence gleaned from these research projects and aimed to address the identified gaps within the community for participation in purposeful and meaningful occupations for persons with serious, persistent mental illness.

Through my research and conversations with mental health consumers, I learned that there existed many individuals who also recognized that the system was not working for them, who

were frustrated by the perception that something different was not likely to happen, and who had ideas of something better for the community-residing mental health consumer.

NISA was created to be an alternative community mental health programme, which initially aimed to provide mental health consumers with the opportunity to participate in meaningful occupation. NISA provided a safe and supportive social environment in which to recover and the opportunity for consumers to decide for themselves what they participated in, and the frequency of their involvement, linking what they did to the larger community. In essence, the NISA programme attempted to correct or remove many of the perceived barriers to participation in occupation identified in the labyrinth study. NISA has since dovetailed into a programme service delivery model (Rebeiro et al 2001), which has been studied since its inception and which continues to be researched on an ongoing basis by an occupational therapist and mental health consumers who participate in ParNorth – the research programme of NISA (Legault & Rebeiro 2001).

The initial considerations for the NISA programme have since been redefined, based on the NISA formative evaluation study, and the findings are shared below. The research continuously shapes and defines both the programme and the role of the occupational therapist within this consumer-governed organization.

APPLICATION OF THE RESEARCH IN PRACTICE

Opportunity, not prescription: the provision of real work opportunity

The initial discussions and planning of NISA considered the major findings learned from the previous research and also the extensive 'system' experience of the consumers who participated at NISA. We knew that we would need to provide opportunity and choice for consumers to participate in real work occupations that were not only personally meaningful to them but also of social value to the larger community. Early participants in the NISA programme recognized that the stigma related to society's perception that mental health consumers were not capable of participating in real work, were incapable of helping themselves or were 'lazy' would need to be addressed as an integral aspect of the NISA programme. Clearly, people were interested in dispelling many of the myths associated with mental illness by what they did at NISA. Thus, from the beginnings, NISA began programmes involving research (the ParNorth unit), publishing an international psychosocial literary journal known as *Open Minds Quarterly*, and undertook the responsibility to receive, repair and donate used computers to persons of need in the community. Each of these programme initiatives has been accorded value by the variety of community partnerships fostered by NISA, and several reciprocal and interdependent partnerships have been developed with not only the formal mental health system, but also the many like-minded community agencies we assist.

The NISA programme has since expanded its occupational programmes to include: making patchwork quilts and blankets for homeless and needy people within our community; an artist's loft that regularly exhibits and sells work in public venues and galleries (indeed, NISA artists have been profiled on the covers of several journals and books); and, most recently, by developing a gift shop located in the lobby of the psychiatric hospital to help address the socioeconomic issues faced by many mental health consumers. Most programmes aim to provide part-time and commission work for NISA members. Many members have also been trained by the occupational therapist to provide solution-focused interventions in the form of the NISA Nightline support telephone service and also in providing peer support to other members while at NISA.

Removal of barriers to inclusion: simplify the labyrinth

A second consideration in developing NISA was ensuring that access to the programme did not constitute a labyrinth and that the previously identified barriers to consumers' access to and

participation in occupational programmes – including referral processes and finances – were removed. NISA subsidizes bus passes to remove finance as a barrier to participation and welcomes any mental health consumer who chooses to self-refer to the programme. People who come to NISA by referral from a professional are informed that they are not obligated to attend – that NISA is a self-directed programme – but if there is something at NISA that interests them, they are welcome to participate when they want and according to their needs.

Levelling of power hierarchies

A third application of the research was to attempt to level any real or perceived hierarchies between consumers and professional staff. This was achieved by the declaration that all members were equal, myself included. All members of NISA had the right to a vote regarding the organizations' decisions, and I sat in *ex officio* capacity during the first year of the Board and in an advisery role thereafter. We all dress casually for work because we recognized that clothing is a sign of material status and a signifier of power. I have an 'open door' policy, and the furniture in my office is arranged to be conducive to conversation, rather than to assessment and interviewing.

Creating a safe and supportive social environment

A further consideration in the development of NISA was the creation of a safe and supportive social environment. NISA takes the provision of a safe environment seriously and, although NISA has very few rules, one concerning courteous behaviour has been in place since the beginning. The courtesy agreement is simple by nature and states that all members have the right to an environment that is respectful of all members and one that is safe both emotionally and physically. Members are encouraged to talk about solutions rather than problems, to focus on their strengths versus perceived weaknesses or shortcomings as persons, and are given feedback and assistance to deal with emotions and issues in a positive and proactive manner. This assistance is initially provided by the occupational therapist and then more generally by NISA members via a peer support network.

APPLICATION OF THE EVIDENCE TO SERVICE DELIVERY AND PRACTICE

The NISA formative evaluation study, which has been conducted by the ParNorth research unit since the beginnings of NISA, has taught us many important lessons about the provision of care, service delivery and practice within a consumer-governed programme. Although many elements of the initial programme were based on the earlier research, the NISA evaluation study taught us ways to define and apply the model better (Rebeiro et al 2001).

There have been many lessons learned from the NISA formative evaluation study (Rebeiro et al 2001). In general, the NISA study has taught us that many of the elements of the environment were appropriate, especially in fostering an environment that was perceived to be safe, which fostered a sense of belonging for members and which encouraged a re-discovery of the self and of one's self-worth. However, what we did not know, but what was made explicit in the NISA study, was the importance of the person's inner healing needs – or 'being' needs – to recovery and to subsequent successful participation in meaningful occupation. The NISA study unveiled the importance of meeting people's 'being, belonging and becoming' needs to recovery – recovery becoming a useful construct for practice and being dependent upon providing opportunity for a full quality life, including participation in occupation. 'Being' needs are about the person, their unqualified humanness and right to exist. 'Being' needs have to do with self-love, self-esteem and a belief in one's own self-worth and right to something better. 'Being' needs are about unconditional acceptance of the person regardless of their past or the 'baggage' they bring with them to NISA.

'Belonging' needs have to do with the environment, about a safe and supportive place to belong and with a feeling that one has been let in and included. 'Becoming' needs are about the individual's right to opportunities for work, for self-fulfilment, for economic security and for participation in meaningful daily roles that are valued in the community.

Through the NISA study, we learned that being and belonging needs in many ways precede becoming needs, or more occupation-based needs. There were many folks who attended NISA, but who were initially unable to participate in any of the programme initiatives. Nonetheless, they indicated a need to be involved in a safe and supportive social environment, such as the one provided at NISA. These individuals tended to be in a stabilizing period of their lives. Those who appeared to benefit most from the occupation-based initiatives were those whose illness was well managed and who appeared to be in the recovery phase of their lives. Previously, I would have thought that I had shortcomings in providing occupational therapy services for clients who chose not to participate in programmes, but the series of focus groups in the NISA formative evaluation study taught me that people who were unable to participate actively in occupations still had many being or internal needs to address. The ongoing research at NISA has shown us that, when people feel accepted for who they are and feel that they have a place to belong, the issues surrounding their active participation in occupation become a next logical step in their recovery process.

HOW RESEARCH EVIDENCE AFFECTED THE AUTHOR'S CLINICAL PRACTICE

These research studies, coupled with my strong commitment to being client-centred, required that I both challenge and eventually change the ways I practised occupational therapy. I learned that there were many mental health consumers who had both a very good appreciation of the systemic problems in mental health services and an appreciation for some of the possible solutions. Research taught me that I had to level any preconceived notions that my education accorded me greater status or claims to expertise. Research enabled me to question practice, assessments and protocols that did not appear to be helpful to clients but which served to perpetuate the system and professional power. Research eventually required me to 'colour outside the lines' of traditional practice by taking risks and engaging in more advocacy at the client, programme and organizational levels (Pike 2001). The following section briefly reviews Shannon Pike's research of my role as the occupational therapist in this consumer-run organization.

Colouring outside the lines of traditional practice

Shannon Pike's (2001) qualitative study of the role of the occupational therapist in NISA helps to highlight the many ways that occupational therapists can practise within non-traditional parameters. Pike conducted in-depth interviews, focus groups and participant observation to collect data on the role of the occupational therapist within a consumer-governed organization. Essentially, Pike illustrated that working in a consumer-run organization requires the occupational therapist to practise differently. In particular, she perceived that the occupational therapist is required to 'colour outside the lines' in terms of not accepting traditional boundaries and learning to question the way things are traditionally done.

According to Pike, *colouring outside the lines* is interpreted as pushing or overrunning traditional boundaries and challenging the barriers that often exist in mental health practice. Specifically, Pike described six elements of practice that helped to define colouring outside the lines and the role of the occupational therapist:

- taking risks
- advocacy at the client, programme and organizational levels
- redefining professionalism
- client-centredness
- establishing common ground
- non-traditional occupational therapy practice.

Taking risks

Taking risks was identified as a way of practising in a consumer-run organization. Taking risks involved practising occupational therapy in a very non-traditional way and included 'going against the grain' of established policies and procedures. For example, the occupational therapist found that, in order to be client-centred, she had to abandon many of the safeguards and boundaries of traditional professional practice in the interest of getting to know clients better and in establishing and securing trusting, effective partnerships. Taking risks also included self-disclosure in order both to gain the trust of the client and to encourage clients to share information about themselves.

Engaging in advocacy at the client, programme and organizational levels

An important role for the occupational therapist in non-traditional practice arenas involves advocacy. Advocacy can take many forms and can occur at many levels. At the clinical level, this may involve advocacy to ensure that the clients' needs are being met (rather than the needs of the referral sources), or it may involve supporting clients in their search for a better medication because their current medication poses a barrier to participation. At the system level, advocacy may include ensuring that clients are active participants in any discussion of programmes, proposed changes or allocation of health resources. At the community level, advocacy for the basic citizenship rights within the community for persons with serious and persistent mental illness might include housing, food or transportation issues, disability support or a clothing allowance. At the level of government, advocacy may involve letter-writing, letters to the editor, publications and conferences to disseminate evidence that supports alternative programmes and theoretical approaches, and lobbying for adequate funding to support alternative partnerships.

Being professional in a 'non-professional' way

Making explicit therapists' professional and personal values helped to realize a unique and reciprocal relationship with participants of the NISA organization. Specifically, Pike's study identified that being human, not fearing to show one's humanness (including weaknesses and acknowledging mistakes), having an equal and reciprocal relationship based on respect, and demonstrating consistency between what is said and what is done, all help to define being professional in a 'non-professional way'.

Client-centredness

Client-centredness is often taken for granted by occupational therapists. In Pike's study, the participants defined client-centredness as being encouraging, assisting or enabling consumers to think for themselves, make informed decisions and exercise choice. Clearly, being client-centred was perceived by participants to be an asset of the occupational therapist at NISA. Being client-centred meant allowing clients to determine their destiny and, using evidence-based occupational therapy, to support their chosen journey.

CONCLUDING THOUGHTS

Tighter restraints on spending, a desire by funding agencies to eliminate hospitalization for persons with mental illness, and subsequent policies and programmes geared to this outcome, leave little room for a profession that aims to assist with quality of life, life satisfaction and active participation in the community. The realities of practice require that occupational therapists are knowledgeable about and use evidence to support their practice. The realities of practice will further demand that occupational therapists maintain current knowledge of the occupational therapy literature and the literature of other disciplines. Therapists need to assume personal and professional responsibility, and begin using evidence to inform and challenge their practice. It is easy to assume that someone else will conduct the research, gather the evidence, and inform practice and theory. It is also easy to assume that all is well – to be complacent with practice and not to challenge the status quo. However, we can no longer work in a professional vacuum. The writing is clearly on the walls that government and funding agencies will fund only

best practices – those that are supported by research.

My personal journey into the world of research has helped me to understand better the relationship between engagement in occupation and mental health. There now exists an evidence base that has not only informed and challenged my practice as an occupational therapist, but has also changed it. Qualitative research has been the means to inform this theoretical base and the manner in which client-centred services may be delivered.

REFERENCES

Cook JV 2001 Qualitative research in occupational therapy: strategies and experiences. Delmar, Albany, NY

Davidson L, Stayner DA, Nickou C et al 2001 Simply to be let in: inclusion as a basis for recovery. Psychiatric Rehabilitation Journal 24:375–388

Deegan P 1992 The independent living movement and people with psychiatric disabilities: taking back control over our own lives. Psychosocial Rehabilitation Journal 15(3):3–19

Estroff SE 1989 Self, identity, and subjective experiences of schizophrenia: in search of the subject. Schizophrenia Bulletin 15:189–196

Goffman E 1963 Stigma: notes on the management of spoiled identity. Simon Schuster, New York

Higgins C 2001 Closing address to delegates. International Association of Psychosocial Rehabilitation Services Conference, Ontario Chapter. Thunder Bay, Ontario

Holstein JA, Gubrium JF 1995 The active interview. Sage, Thousand Oaks, CA

Jorgenson DL 1989 Participant observation: a methodology for human studies. Sage, Newbury Park, CA

Leete E 1989 How I perceive and manage my illness. Schizophrenia Bulletin 15:197–200

Legault E, Rebeiro KL 2001 Occupation-as-means to mental health: a single case study. American Journal of Occupational Therapy 55:90–96

Lincoln YS, Guba EG 1985 Naturalistic inquiry. Sage, Newbury Park, CA

McCracken G 1988 The long interview. Sage, Newbury Park, CA

Morgan DL 1988 Focus groups as qualitative research. Sage, Newbury Park, CA

Pike SE 2001 Colouring outside the lines: defining the role of the occupational therapist in a consumer-run organization. University of Western Ontario, London, Ontario

Rebeiro KL 1997 Opportunity, not prescription: an exploratory study of the experience of occupational engagement. University of Western Ontario, London, Ontario

Rebeiro KL 1998 Occupation-as-means to mental health: a review of the literature and a call to research. Canadian Journal of Occupational Therapy 66:12–19

Rebeiro KL 1999 The labyrinth of community mental health: in search of meaningful occupation. Psychiatric Rehabilitation Journal 23:143–152

Rebeiro KL 2000 Client perspectives on occupational therapy practice: are we truly client-centred? Canadian Journal of Occupational Therapy 67:7–14

Rebeiro KL 2001a Occupational terminology interactive dialogue: the model of occupational spin-off. Journal of Occupational Science 8:33–34

Rebeiro KL 2001b In order to make a difference: a research journey. In: Cook JV (ed) Qualitative research in occupational therapy: strategies and experiences. Delmar, Albany, NY; pp. 133–155

Rebeiro KL, Allen J 1998 Voluntarism as occupation. Canadian Journal of Occupational Therapy 65:279–285

Rebeiro KL, Cook JV 1999 Opportunity, not prescription: an exploratory study of the experience of occupational engagement. Canadian Journal of Occupational Therapy 66:176–187

Rebeiro KL, Day DG, Semeniuk B et al 2001 Northern Initiative for Social Action: an occupation-based mental health program. American Journal of Occupational Therapy 55:493–500

Townsend E 1998 Good intentions overruled: a critique of empowerment in the routine organization of mental health services. University of Toronto Press, Toronto

Townsend E, Rebeiro KL 2001 Open forum: Canada's joint position statement on evidence-based occupational therapy. OTNow Jan/Feb:9–11

Whyte WF (ed) 1991 Participatory action research. Sage, Newbury Park, CA

FURTHER READING

Cook JV 2001 Qualitative research in occupational therapy: strategies and experiences. Delmar, Albany, NY

Holstein JA, Gubrium JF 1995 The active interview. Sage, Thousand Oaks, CA

Lincoln YS, Guba EG 1985 Naturalistic inquiry. Sage, Newbury Park, CA

Townsend E 1998 Good intentions overruled: a critique of empowerment in the routine organization of mental health services. University of Toronto Press, Toronto

9

Using a multiple case-study research design to develop an understanding of clinical expertise in physical therapy

Jan Gwyer   Gail Jensen   Laurita Hack
Katherine Shepard

OVERVIEW

Proponents of evidence-based practice acknowledge the importance of clinical expertise. However, this compelling concept is not easily defined, nor has it been subjected to rigorous research in medicine or the rehabilitation sciences. As a result, clinical expertise has been assigned less value than other forms of 'scientific' evidence. In this chapter, Jan Gwyer, Gail Jensen, Laurita Hack and Katherine Shepard describe how they used a qualitative multiple case-study approach to investigate the nature of clinical expertise in a diversity of physiotherapy practice areas. Based on their findings, these authors developed a theoretical model of expert practice in physical therapy, the components of which illuminate how clinical expertise is acquired and sustained. The research findings constitute evidence to support physiotherapy theory development and client-centred practice, and to develop educational strategies that promote evidence-based practice in rehabilitation that is grounded in the broad definition of evidence needed to address clients' needs in a relevant and effective manner.

C.C.

INTRODUCTION

Many practitioners are fascinated, like us, with the question, 'What does it mean to acquire expertise?' This chapter describes our journey of investigative work into dimensions of expertise in physical therapy. We will highlight the findings of a qualitative research study that used a multiple case-study approach, and how these findings led to the development of a theoretical model of expert practice in physical therapy.

Dr Jules Rothstein, writing in the foreword to our book on expertise (Jensen et al 1999), reminds us that expertise is a compelling yet complex concept for health professionals:

'Science can be used to study expertise, and a variety of research methods can be used to understand how experts function and how to enhance practice by mimicking some of their behaviors. But first we must define what it means to be an expert. We should realize that factors such as the numbers of courses taken, the number of continuing education courses taught, or reverence of colleagues do not really identify an expert. In my view, true expertise means a practitioner can be something better, and data exists to support this contention' (p. xviii).

Thus, expertise is much more than experience, technical skill or problem-solving ability. What, then, accounts for expertise in physical therapy?

WHAT PROMPTED THE RESEARCH: BEGINNING THE JOURNEY

Our interest in exploring expertise grew from our clinical experiences. Two of us were working in the same clinical setting and had repeated conversations about the qualities we believed helped define 'master clinicians'. These conversations were always in the context of actual patient care. We were fortunate to be working in a practice that had attracted several clinicians whom we believed demonstrated expertise. We were able to watch them with patients and we recognized that they were consistently able to display characteristics that we did not see in novice or mediocre clinicians. We saw clinicians who spent time listening, who spent time in teaching, who were truly engaged with patients. These clinicians enjoyed their work and seemed energized by it. They were curious and constantly sought more information about patient care. They seemed to have positive outcomes with patients, including high return rates and good cooperation with the plan of care.

We knew that not all therapists behaved in this manner. We knew that students and novice clinicians had different patterns of behaviour. They appeared to spend their time in different ways, with less emphasis on listening and teaching. We agreed that we had seen colleagues with many years' experience who did not display these positive behaviours, who had high no-show rates, who spent far less time with their patients, and who seemed much more task-oriented in their care. We also knew colleagues who expressed boredom and dissatisfaction with practising physical therapy.

In addition, there were many pressures in the healthcare system that discouraged the behaviours that we associated with quality care. We saw increasing demands for productivity, a lack of clarity about what constituted good outcomes, increasing controls over care by non-clinicians, and increasing attempts to reduce healthcare costs by reducing access to physical therapy. These factors have continued to grow over the past 12 years.

For these reasons, we were motivated to understand the differences among the clinicians with whom we worked. Many questions arose as we continued our discussions. Why do some people acquire expertise, but not others? Are there differences across the range of years of experience? What are these differences? Are there differences across clinical specialty areas? How do people who seem to be 'experts' acquire their expertise? Is their clinical reasoning different from that of other therapists? What, exactly, is mastery or expertise? We became committed to exploring ways to answer these questions.

We recognized immediately that traditional quantitative research methods would not lead us to a better understanding of these issues. These were not issues that lent themselves to experimental intervention. Quantitative descriptive techniques, such as surveys, were also inadequate for our purposes. We determined that we needed to use a qualitative methodology because it would allow us fully to explore the phenomenon of expertise in physical therapy in actual practice settings.

Our first imperative was to refine our questions. We carried out several preliminary studies (Jensen et al 1990, 1992) that used observation and analysis of patient–therapist interaction videotapes to generate themes that explored the differences between therapists with less experience and those with more experience. These studies confirmed that novice clinicians and experienced clinicians behaved in different ways in the provision of patient care. Through these studies we developed a conceptual framework that helped us to identify successive steps in our research process and to focus our subsequent research on questions that had to do with expertise itself.

WHY THE METHODS CHOSEN FIT THE RESEARCH PURPOSE

Understanding the phenomenon of expertise

Much of the research in the study of expertise has emphasized the central importance of cognition and the mental processing skills of the expert. This first generation of expert theory included clinical problem-solving studies in medicine, where experts and novices were compared to see how they represented and solved problems. A second generation of theoretical work linked research participants' clinical reasoning skills to their knowledge base. Here differences were seen in the way the experts and novices organized their knowledge. Experts had a specific recall of meaningful relationships and patterns, and a structure to the knowledge they used as well as a problem-solving strategy (Ericsson 1996, Ericsson & Smith 1991, Higgs & Jones 2000). We were very interested in understanding more fully what experts actually do in practice, including the experiences and meanings that are part of the context and interactions of everyday practice in physical therapy.

Our investigative aim was consistent with a conception of expertise that is multidimensional. Such a concept goes beyond a focus on knowledge or skill acquisition, or an individual's mental processing, to consider who the person is, how they perceive themselves, their professional development, and their interactions and performance in practice (Benner et al 1996, Higgs & Jones 2000, Higgs & Titchen 2001, Mattingly & Flemming 1994).

Qualitative case-study design

To obtain this greater understanding of the expert and expert practice, we had to 'center [ourselves] in the *clinical world*, in the eye of the storm' (Miller & Crabtree 2000, p. 611). We wanted to understand and document the uniqueness and complexity of expert practice. To do that, we employed a qualitative case-study design. While some researchers would argue that case-study design is a research process (Yin 1994), others would define a case as a unit of study, 'a case of something' (Stake 2000). Merriam, in her recent text on case-study research, defines a case as 'a bounded system – a case as a thing, a single entity, a unit around which there are boundaries' (Merriam 1998, p. 27). In addition, Merriam describes qualitative case studies as being characterized as being particularistic, descriptive and heuristic. In our research we wanted to explore the *particular* situation or phenomenon of expert practice in physical therapy. We wanted to understand how expert clinicians thought, reasoned, made decisions, what meanings they attached to their professional lives and what the important markers were during their growth from novice to expert. We also wanted to *describe* expert practice as richly and fully as possible using the voices and experiences of expert therapists. The data-rich cases could then be used for theory development across the clinical areas of investigation. We were intent upon enhancing our understanding of expert practice as well as discovering new meaning through a *heuristic* approach where the design, meanings and actions of expert practice are explored in the clinician's natural setting.

The qualitative case-study design also provided us a way to 'fence in' or bound the study. The case-study design provides a structure within which the four of us could each study one clinical area in physical therapy practice. The case-study design also assists in setting the boundaries for what is part of the investigation and what is not. We were interested in gaining insight into experts' professional development and in understanding their practice as experienced in the natural setting – the clinic. A multiple case-study design gave us a template or action plan for organizing our data collection across the four researchers (Merriam 1998).

Each of us collected data in one clinical area: geriatrics, neurology, orthopaedics or paediatrics. We studied three therapists in each of the four clinical areas for a total of 12 therapists. An essential question in any case-study design is: 'What is the "unit of analysis"?'. We began the study by collecting data on each therapist representing a single case, written as a *case report*. As we continued to gather data on the second and third therapists, we began to look across the case reports of the three therapists in our clinical area as well as the therapists in the other clinical areas. For each of the clinical areas we wrote a *composite case study* that represented a description of expert practice. At this point our unit of analysis was now the composite description of expert practice across the three therapists. A final component of the *multiple case-study design* was the development of grounded theory or theory building (Fig. 9.1).

DESCRIPTION OF THE RESEARCH PROCESS

Involving clinicians as participants in the study

The 12 clinicians involved in the study were identified as experts through a peer nomination

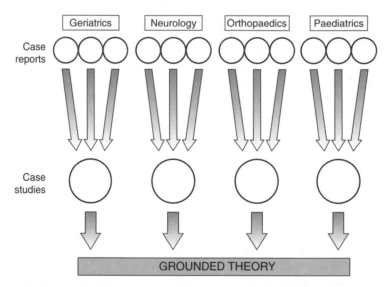

Figure 9.1 Multiple case-study design. (After Jensen et al 1999, with kind permission of Butterworth-Heinemann.)

process. Officers of the American Physical Therapy Association (APTA) clinical specialty sections were contacted to provide nominations of expert practitioners based on criteria developed during previous work on clinician expertise (Schmidt et al 1990). These criteria were that participants:

- had 7 years or more of clinical practice
- were involved in direct patient care at least 50% of the time
- had completed formal or informal advanced work in a clinical specialty area
- were people to whom the nominator would refer a patient with complications or would select for care of a family member.

Final selection was based on those clinicians who had received the highest number of criterion-based nominations from the officers and who were geographically closest to the investigator who was studying that clinical specialty area. Institutional review board approval was obtained from each investigator's academic institution as well as from each hospital setting where some of the clinicians practised.

Data collection methods

Methods used to gather data included on-site non-participant observations, a series of in-depth interviews, videotapes of patient evaluation and treatment sessions, and a review of documents such as patient records and patient teaching materials. The interviews took two forms. The first was the professional development interview in which structured tasks were used to stimulate the clinician's recall of his or her professional 'journey' (Box 9.1).

The second interview was the response to the patient videotape interview during which clinicians were asked a number of questions regarding their knowledge and clinical reasoning processes while viewing their performance with patients (Box 9.2).

Data were gathered from each therapist working with at least three patients over a single episode of care. 'Episodes of care' were defined as all physical therapy visits provided for each

patient during a 'single episode', or up to 3 months of care for patients with chronic impairments. Data were collected on each clinician until data saturation was achieved.

Data reduction and analyses

The sequence of data reduction and analysis was organized around the four major cognitive process phases that Morse (1994) identified as being used in managing qualitative data. This process is displayed in Figure 9.2. In the first phase – 'comprehending' – data were gathered, triangulated and coded according to the open and axial coding process identified by Strauss & Corbin (1998). Members of the investigation team who had not been involved in data collection reviewed the coded data. Subsequent to lengthy discussions on data content and intent, decision rules were created to ensure that the final coding

---

Box 9.1 Professional development interview guide

- Each participant's resumé was reviewed and listed in categories on note cards (e.g. education, professional associations). The participant was then asked to sort the note cards into three piles, from most important to least important effect on their development of expertise.
- After these categories had been sorted, the therapists were asked to talk about each of the events in the categories. Why have you grouped these together? What is meaningful about this course (or person, experience, etc.)?
- How has your knowledge of physical therapy changed over time? How has your knowledge of your specialty area changed over time? Describe an example. To what do you attribute these changes?
- What aspects of your clinical knowledge have changed the most over time? What are the sources of your clinical knowledge?
- How did you acquire your present decision-making style? How has this style changed over the years? Describe an example. What do you believe accounts for these changes?
- What do you consider to be milestones in your learning that have led to your becoming the clinician you are today?
- What advice would you give new graduates wanting to become experts in your area of practice?

Box 9.2 Interview guide for debriefing interviews

- What were you thinking about as you completed your evaluation with the patient? What is your diagnosis? What evidence did you use? How do you know what information to focus on? Where did you learn that? Where will you go next?
- Talk about what is going on with this patient. What is your prognosis? How did you reach that conclusion? What evidence did you use? How did you know to use that evidence? Where did you learn that?
- Talk to me about your most difficult problem with this patient. How did you identify the problem? What evidence did you use? What was your strategy for solving the problem? How did you learn to do this?
- Describe how you went about making clinical decisions with this patient? What is your approach? Describe an example as we go through the tape.
- Is this process of making a decision different for you now, compared with when you were a novice clinician? What are the differences?
- What do you think your best patient care skills are? What knowledge do you draw upon as you execute these skills? (Look at video for specific examples.)
- How do you know you have been effective in your evaluation and treatment of this patient?
- What would you tell a student about how to go about decision-making in this patient care environment? Would what you tell a student differ from what you actually do? How would it be different and why?

scheme contained independent and mutually exclusive coding categories.

In the second phase – 'synthesizing' – case reports were written on each clinician following a common categorical outline, obtained from the axial coding scheme. Thus, each case report contained six components: (1) clinician's personal history and professional development milestones; (2) identification of the types and sources of knowledge used by the clinician in clinical practice; (3) description of the clinician's clinical reasoning processes; (4) description of the clinician's philosophy of practice; (5) description of the clinician's disposition, values and beliefs; and (6) identification of the clinician's physical therapy skills.

In the third phase – 'theorizing' – the investigative team read each of the four clinical specialty area case reports. Using a strategy described by Yin (1994) as 'pattern matching and explanation building', a single, composite case study was written for each clinical specialty area.

During the fourth phase – 'recontextualizing' – the four case reports were analysed for common themes (Shepard et al 1999). These common themes became the basis for identification of the core dimensions of expert practice in physical therapy (Fig. 9.3).

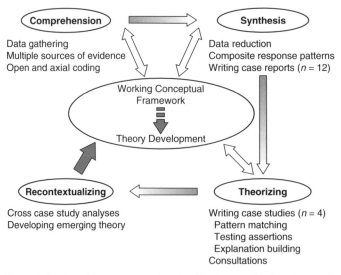

Figure 9.2 Cognitive processes involved in the qualitative data analysis. (After Jensen et al 1999, with kind permission of Butterworth-Heinemann. Originally adapted from Morse 1994.)

Strategies to ensure the integrity of the research

The following techniques were used to ensure that the qualitative data obtained and the subsequent data analyses were dependable and credible (Creswell 1997):

1. Prolonged engagement and focused observation in the field.
2. Triangulation of data using multiple data sources, multiple methods and multiple investigators.
3. Rich, thick descriptions. The data are presented in the form of lengthy direct quotations from the clinicians participating in the study. These types of data, known as low-inference data, allow the reader to determine whether the investigator's interpretations are true to the content and intent of the data.
4. Member checks. Each clinician case report was returned to the clinician to review and, if necessary, revise to ensure accuracy in content and meaning.
5. Use of three consultants unconnected with the study or the practice of physical therapy. These consultants, who were nationally known university professors skilled in qualitative research, medical expertise and

decision-making processes, reviewed and provided comments on the case report content and interpretations and emerging theory development. As a result of their consultation, we returned to the field to gather additional data for verification.
6. Peer review at each stage of developing the case report and case studies. This peer evaluation was instrumental in challenging each investigator as to potential blind spots, inconsistencies and biases that crept into the writing.

In relation to the participants, we have been asked various forms of the same question that might be summarized as, 'How expert were your "experts"?' and 'How representative are they of most physical therapists in a diversity of clinical settings?'. In providing detailed descriptions of each participant's case we hoped that consumers of this research would be able to judge these dimensions for themselves. We also learnt from our participants that an expert does not perform with expertise 100% of the time in a complex practice. These clinicians expressed genuine humility during the study and were comfortable discussing what they did not understand in their practice and reflecting on the patient problems they could not address effectively. As a result of this work, we feel confident in describing each expert clinician as a physical therapist with a core philosophy of practice, arising from the dimensions of multidimensional knowledge, collaborative clinical reasoning, movement and practice, and virtuous practice that consistently guide their practice. These findings were used to develop a theoretical model of expert practice (Fig. 9.3).

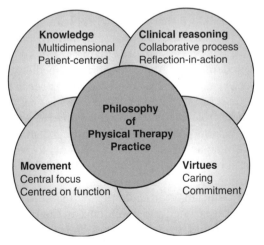

Figure 9.3 Core dimensions of expert practice in physical therapy. (After Jensen et al 1999, with kind permission of Butterworth-Heinemann.)

THE RESEARCH FINDINGS: DIMENSIONS OF EXPERT PRACTICE IN PHYSICAL THERAPY

Multidimensional knowledge base

The participants had acquired an amazingly broad and deep content knowledge to support their specialty practice, and through the interviews the participants were able to describe the development of this multidimensional knowledge base. Early in their careers they developed two important skills: (1) the ability to identify various sources of information by which their knowledge base could be expanded, and (2) the ability to organize and transform their knowledge through reflection on their clinical experience.

The expert clinicians demonstrated a continual desire to enhance their knowledge, and demonstrated initiative and determination in finding sources of knowledge useful to them. Some found immediate holes in their professional education and began searching for sources to fill these gaps. All found clinical mentors whose practice they respected and who agreed to facilitate their learning in the clinical setting. These mentors had greatly expanded the participants' sources of knowledge, introducing them to continuing and graduate education opportunities and to interdisciplinary colleagues. During the early years of practice, each participant reported learning about the importance of the patient as a source of information. This lesson was sometimes learned the hard way, requiring significant self-discipline in learning to listen carefully. Each participant found their clinical reasoning skills to be greatly enhanced as they gained the ability to hear and incorporate patients' understanding and knowledge. This knowledge – and the answers that the patient sought – became the focus of the physical therapy assessment and intervention. Over time, the emphasis on patient-focused care led them to master knowledge of psychological development, family and social systems, and patient advocacy in private and public arenas. This broadened, multidimensional knowledge base enabled these expert clinicians to gain a much fuller understanding of their role as physical therapists than that expressed by novices in our earlier research studies.

As these clinicians experienced the valuable source of knowledge inherent in each patient encounter, they began the process of transforming their knowledge base in significant ways. Each patient encounter provided evidence to support or refute treatment or diagnostic decisions, and the participants began a process of reflection on their actions that made a significant difference to their practice. This process appeared to be especially intense in the early years of their practice, or when they changed specialty areas. However, the clinicians involved in this study continued to use each patient encounter as an opportunity to learn and to restructure what they considered to be of central importance for a patient with a certain diagnosis or movement dysfunction. Mentors also facilitated the participants' reflection on practice by guiding them through patient problems and encouraging them to think critically. Throughout this process the clinical knowledge and expertise the clinicians developed was situated in practice and centred on patients, thereby enhancing retrieval of information and self-reflection. These meta-cognitive skills were refined through the guidance of mentors in both the clinical setting and the academic setting during graduate work.

Collaborative clinical reasoning

The participants consistently identified the patient as a valuable source of knowledge, so it was not surprising to find that they preferred a collaborative clinical reasoning process, one that intensely involved the patient or the patient's family. The patients' medical diagnosis was a supplemental piece of information, only generally guiding the therapist's data collection. The patient's statements of problems, goals or concerns more typically directed the initial definition of the therapist's diagnosis. Once the patient's problems had been understood by both the therapist and the patient, an intense process of prioritizing solutions was engaged upon by the patient and the therapist. These expert clinicians conveyed a deep sense that patients are in charge of their care and that the clinician's role is to empower the patient to achieve their goals successfully. They encouraged students to adopt an approach in which patients focus and direct their own care, rather than their healthcare practitioners.

The clinicians participating in this study displayed proficiency and confidence in their clinical reasoning and in approaching complex patient situations, and considered that these challenging situations stimulated the most learning. They also displayed confidence in their ability constantly to evaluate the patient in order to correct a mistake in either diagnosis or treatment decisions, and demonstrated their willingness to admit their mistakes and correct them quickly. This confidence enabled them to take risks in their clinical decision-making, and this was a highly valued ability. Some of the clinicians felt that the optimal benefit for the patient was not attained without incorporating such risks into their practice. They trusted their tacit or craft knowledge, and used it in making intuitive decisions about patient care. 'Function', as this was defined by the patient, formed the core of a framework used in establishing patient care goals. This goal-setting process required clinicians to use their in-depth specialty knowledge when considering normal and achievable function.

Movement and practice

The skilled facilitation of controlled movement is the core of physical therapists' practice, and the participants demonstrated a grace and fluidity in this psychomotor skill that, as physical therapy investigators, we found impressive. The clinicians used movement to connect to their patients for various purposes: to gain both quantitative and qualitative data about the patient's movements, to guide or stabilize the patient during treatment, and to communicate reassurance or praise. Our understanding of these deceptively familiar movements was enhanced by the therapists' reflections on their videotaped sessions with patients. During these debriefing interviews we confirmed the purpose of their movements, which appeared to flow seamlessly from evaluation to treatment to teaching. The clinicians identified intuitive movements used during treatment sessions. These were described as movements that they did not plan and that they could not explain before performing them.

Assessment and observation of movement requires a deep and complex understanding of normal and abnormal movement. This knowledge enabled the expert clinicians to analyse movement efficiently and effectively. They took advantage of all opportunities to observe their patients, balancing their time observing the patient with that spent touching the patient, because they consistently believed that everything changes after the therapist touches the patient. Their focus was intense, allowing them to analyse movement while simultaneously talking with and listening to patients. They considered their hands – and in some cases their entire bodies – to be important evaluative tools and they relied heavily on what they learned and understood about the patient through use of their hands. These clinicians demonstrated a finely tuned kinesthetic awareness of what patients were communicating through their bodies. They could recall with confidence how specific patients looked and felt when moving, even over long time periods between visits. How did these clinicians develop such refined movement and movement analysis skills? Most stated that their skills improved through reflection on their intense, deliberate and focused practice of treatment techniques. Mentors also assisted them to refine their movement skills by encouraging them to concentrate on the information they were gaining both through their hands and through observation.

Virtuous practice

As we each developed the case studies in the four specialty areas, we identified a shared admiration for the clinicians as people, and their 'virtuous' characteristics emerged as an important dimension of expertise. Several of the participants identified professional moral dilemmas that caused them to make tough choices that had personal and professional consequences. The commitment to clinical practice that characterized their careers served to provide the resolve and ability to make reasoned ethical and moral decisions in these situations.

Their commitment to patients served to motivate these therapists to pursue the other dimensions of the model of expertise, and this could prove quite demanding on their lives. We observed that each clinician demonstrated a deep and sincere value for patients that inspired not only their quest for knowledge and clinical reasoning skills, but also a belief that patient advocacy was an integral component of their role, requiring of them a considerable expenditure of time and energy. Commitment to patients was a central feature of all the clinician cases. It derived from the therapists' sense of caring and compassion, and was reinforced by their strong desire to learn and develop their clinical competence. We identified the following virtuous behaviours as characteristic of an expert clinician:

- non-judgemental approaches to collaborative problem-solving
- embracing responsibility for patient care that often expanded to include advocating for patients, for example ensuring that patients received the resources they needed
- honest discussions with patients when misdiagnoses or other evaluation or treatment mistakes were made
- personal (physical and emotional) commitment to individual patient care – these clinicians set high standards for their performance in terms of doing, to the best of their ability, what best served the patient
- assuming responsibility for identifying and reporting any unethical behaviours of colleagues and other professionals.

Philosophy of practice

The study findings provide evidence to support defining physical therapy expertise in terms of the four dimensions of: a multidimensional and accessible knowledge base; a collaborative and efficient clinical reasoning process; the focused use of movement; and the virtues of caring and compassion for patients. As each of the clinicians developed and refined these four dimensions of practice through reflection on their career experience, their philosophy of practice emerged. The specialty area clearly influenced the expression of the participants' philosophy of practice, but consistent themes emerged that were common to all the cases. These themes included:

- value for the patient as the person in charge of his or her health care
- value for human life regardless of the disability
- value for functional treatment goals defined by the patient

- belief in the benefit of physical therapy
- willingness to serve as a patient advocate
- a sense of moral obligation to maintain a high standard of practice.

CONTRIBUTIONS OF QUALITATIVE RESEARCH ON EXPERTISE IN PHYSICAL THERAPY

Development of evidence-based practice

The development of evidence-based practice has expanded to include 'the integration of best research evidence *with* clinical expertise and patient values' (Sackett et al 2000, p. 1). This broadened definition acknowledges the importance of the clinician's ability to use past experience to make clinical decisions, and to identify patients' preferences and expectations for care. This research on expertise in physical therapy supports the importance of the experiential knowledge of expert clinicians as a source of evidence for physical therapy practice, and strengthens the argument that expert opinion in physical therapy is a valid source of evidence upon which practice can be based.

While included in the definition of evidence-based practice, the 'hierarchy of evidence' (see Ch. 1) places expert opinion on the lowest rung of the ladder (Tonelli 1999). Perhaps this position is the result of the belief that clinical expertise is poorly defined, lacks objectivity and cannot be quantified. This study addresses some of these concerns by providing an in-depth description of expertise in physical therapy. The theoretical model that evolved from the study findings can be used to frame further analysis of expert practice in physical therapy, and employed as a basis for the documentation and discussion, within the profession, of the contributions of expert opinion to evidence-based practice. Quantitative research approaches – higher on the hierarchy of evidence – test the efficacy of physical therapy knowledge across a diversity of practitioners and clinical settings. Qualitative research approaches provide rich descriptions of how expert clinicians seek out, critique and use evidence in making diagnostic and intervention decisions in the 'real' world of clinical practice. The research findings also highlight how this essential knowledge is transferred from expert practitioners to students and their colleagues.

Physical therapist education

These research findings suggest that there is a need for professional education to be rooted in clinical practice, and a need to involve clinicians in teaching the integration of patient care skills with relevant scientific knowledge in providing optimal patient service. In addition, such clinicians would promote the importance of lifelong learning and the reflection on practice that results in deliberative, moral action. The research findings also suggest that students should be encouraged to use the following strategies when learning in clinical settings:

- Value both the clinical instructor *and* the patient as sources of knowledge.
- Listen carefully to the patient and seek an understanding of the meanings that patients attribute to health and illness.
- Develop both cognitive skills *and* the ability to observe keenly and use touch skilfully to facilitate patients' functional movements. Effective integration of these intellectual and practical skills requires both intense focus and continuity of practice.
- Seek out and value a wide spectrum of sources of knowledge, including the 'lived experience of the patient' (Edwards 2001), and enjoy the challenge of embedding this new knowledge in everyday practice.
- Attend to the clinical instructors' process of 'thinking out loud' as they identify and solve patient problems and thus learn to reflect in practice.

Expert clinicians can contribute in significant ways to both the professional education of physical therapy students and the mentoring of novice practitioners. Through their intense self-evaluation and reflection on practice, they can identify more clearly the tacit components of their practice

and thereby effectively facilitate reflective practice in others. There is a need to identify these expert clinicians in our profession and encourage them to become role models and mentors for the next generation of physical therapists. Students and novice practitioners would benefit from being encouraged to develop mentor relationships throughout their careers. Such relationships facilitate the sharing of knowledge and expertise, and are an important component of lifelong learning.

The participants considered patient education to be an important component of their practice. Often the success of the whole patient interaction rested on the clinician's ability to teach the patient and family successfully. Thus, students need knowledge of – and skills in – effective teaching and learning, as well as an understanding of the difficult process of influencing health behaviours. Finally, our novice colleagues need to be supported in incorporating into their everyday practice the virtues of caring, compassion and commitment. They need to observe practitioners who demonstrate these virtues in practice and be challenged to emulate them.

Client-centred practice

The recent shift in evidence-based practice from 'de-emphasizing' toward 'integrating' alternative forms of clinical knowledge and reasoning represents an acknowledgement of the gap that has existed between research and practice. This gap can be bridged by clinicians incorporating patient values, experience and preferences into clinical decision-making (Tonelli 1999). Our research findings demonstrate that clinical decision-making entails different types of knowledge and reasoning processes, and that understanding the perspective of the patient is necessary in making clinical judgements. Collaboration with patients was a central element of the participants' day to day practice. This patient-centred focus is a fundamental component of what Benner et al (1996) describe as deliberative clinical judgement. They argue that clinical judgements cannot be made without understanding the patients' interpretation of their situation and by integrating both professional expertise and patient knowledge in the decision-making process.

CONCLUDING THOUGHTS

The participants in this study demonstrated complex clinical reasoning skills focused on the unique circumstances of each individual patient while simultaneously recalling pertinent outcome information from their 'databank' of previous similar cases. Acquisition of this type of 'databank' or experiential information requires in-depth involvement with patients over time in order that clinicians can thoroughly assess and critique treatment or programme outcomes, and in turn use that information to benefit subsequent patients. Practice models that promote the consultative or supervisory roles of physical therapists result in patient care being substantially delegated to another provider, for example physical therapy assistants. Under these circumstances, the physical therapist is denied the opportunity to learn from the therapeutic relationship developed over time between the patient and therapist, and from the changes in patient outcomes resulting from the clinical or education interventions provided.

The development of expertise requires a considerable commitment in terms of resources and time on the part of both the clinician and the facility or clinic administration. In reality, both resources and time are scarce commodities in the current healthcare system. However, in order to develop the clinical expertise demonstrated by the study participants, physical therapists need time with patients and colleagues, and time for reflection and to consult the literature. These research findings point to the need for clinicians and administrators to acknowledge the essential nature of this contextual learning and facilitate the acquisition of clinical expertise by collaboratively employing creative time management and resource allocation strategies into everyday practice.

Experts are likely to be recognized as outstanding by their peers in terms of knowledge, skills and performance (Benner et al 1996). However, the acquisition of expertise is not a static process and requires continual growth, reflection and lifelong learning. Expertise has been a difficult concept to define, primarily because this kind of knowledge is usually taken for granted and tacit, and therefore less available for acquisition by novice practitioners, or used as 'evidence' to support practice. This study demonstrates the contribution that qualitative research can make to the explication of complex concepts such as clinical expertise and to the development of theoretical models upon which further research can be based. Such research is needed to track the development of clinical expertise during the course of a practitioner's career and to investigate whether clinical expertise can be correlated with more effective patient care outcomes.

The profession needs to be able systematically to define and facilitate physical therapy clinical expertise so that we can both justify practice in individual patient situations and maintain high standards of practice through critical review of the profession's knowledge base. Clinical experts engage in critique, debate, contestation and validation of 'practice knowledge' with colleagues, other disciplines and researchers (Titchen & Ersser 2001), and as such are the key to the development of new knowledge within a profession. Under these circumstances, 'rather than the lowest form of empirical evidence, expert opinion could easily be viewed as the highest form of clinical judgement' (Tonelli 1999, p. 1190).

REFERENCES

Benner P, Tanner CA, Chesla CA 1996 Expertise in nursing practice. Springer, New York

Creswell J 1997 Qualitative inquiry and research design. Sage, Thousand Oaks, CA

Edwards I 2001 Clinical reasoning in three different fields of physiotherapy – a qualitative case study approach. PhD dissertation, University of South Australia, Adelaide

Ericsson KA (ed) 1996 The road to excellence. Lawrence Erlbaum, Mahwah, NJ

Ericsson KA, Smith J (eds) 1991 Toward a general theory of expertise. Cambridge University Press, New York

Higgs J, Jones M (eds) 2000 Clinical reasoning in the health professions. 2nd edn. Butterworth-Heinemann, Oxford

Higgs J, Titchen A 2001 Practice knowledge and expertise in the health professions. Butterworth-Heinemann, Oxford

Jensen GM, Shepard KF, Hack LM 1990 The novice versus the experienced clinician: insights into the work of the physical therapist. Physical Therapy 70:314–323

Jensen GM, Shepard KF, Gwyer J, Hack LM 1992 Attribute dimensions that distinguish master and novice physical therapy clinicians in orthopedic settings. Physical Therapy 72:711–722

Jensen GM, Gwyer J, Hack L, Shepard K 1999 Expertise in physical therapy practice. Butterworth-Heinemann, Boston, MA

Mattingly C, Fleming MH 1994 Clinical reasoning. FA Davis, Philadelphia, PA

Merriam S 1998 Qualitative research and case study applications in education. Jossey-Bass, San Francisco, CA

Miller W, Crabtree B 2000 Clinical research. In: Denzin N, Lincoln Y (eds) Handbook of qualitative research. Sage, Thousand Oaks, CA; pp. 607–631

Morse J (ed) 1994 Critical issues in qualitative research methods. Sage, Thousand Oaks, CA

Sackett DL, Straus SE, Richardson WS, Rosenberg WM, Haynes RB 2000 How to practice and teach evidence-based medicine. Churchill-Livingstone, New York

Schmidt HG, Norman GR, Boshuizen HP 1990 A cognitive perspective on medical expertise: theory and implications. Academic Medicine 65:611–621

Shepard KF, Hack L, Gwyer J, Jensen G 1999 Grounded theory approach to describing the phenomenon of expert practice in physical therapy. Qualitative Health Research 9(6):747–758

Stake R 2000 Case studies. In: Denzin N, Lincoln Y (eds) Handbook of qualitative research. 2nd edn. Sage, Thousand Oaks, CA; pp. 435–454

Strauss A, Corbin J 1998 Basics of qualitative research: grounded theory procedures and techniques. Sage, Thousand Oaks, CA

Titchen A, Ersser S 2001 Explicating, creating and validating professional craft knowledge. In: Higgs J, Titchen A (eds) Practice knowledge and expertise in the health professions. Butterworth-Heinemann, Oxford; pp. 48–56

Tonelli MR 1999 In defense of expert opinion. Academic Medicine 74:1187–1192

Yin R 1994 Case study research design and methods. 2nd edn. Sage, Thousand Oaks, CA

Exploring views and perceptions of evidence-based practice: influencing practice

Michael Curtin   Emily Jaramazovic

KEY POINTS

mixing qualitative and quantitative methods; triangulation; questionnaire design; using evidence in practice

OVERVIEW

Chapter 10 provides the last illustration of research designed to generate qualitative evidence with which to inform practice. Michael Curtin and Emily Jaramazovic describe a study that mixed qualitative and quantitative methods of research to explore the perspectives of evidence-based practice held by occupational therapists in the south of England. The authors demonstrate how qualitative research was used to ensure the relevance and usefulness of a subsequent quantitative survey, and how the evidence generated by these mixed methods served, in turn, to inform and influence practice. Through the example of their research, they prompt consideration of the ways in which research evidence can infiltrate and influence practice, thereby ensuring that clients receive interventions that are both effective and appropriate to their needs.

K.H.

INTRODUCTION

This chapter is separated into two distinct but linked sections. The first section details the methodology used in research investigating the views and opinions of evidence-based practice (EBP) held by occupational therapists working in the south of England. A detailed description of methodology is included in this chapter, both to demonstrate how systematic and rigorous procedures of multitriangulation can enhance the reliability and value of research, and also to provide an example of how two different research approaches might be combined.

The second section of the chapter presents one way in which the findings of the research were used to influence practice. The findings were used as the basis for a one-day workshop, and a summary of the group discussions is presented. This is included to encourage readers to consider ways in which they can work with their colleagues to develop more evidence-based ways of working.

METHODOLOGICAL DETAILS

BACKGROUND TO THE RESEARCH

Despite research that had been conducted investigating health professionals' views on EBP (Barnard & Wiles 2001, Closs & Lewin 1998, Cusick & McCluskey 2000, Dubouloz et al 1999, Pringle 1999, Upton 1999), none was found that specifically identified the opinions of occupational therapists working in England.

The aims of the research conducted by the authors was to identify the views and perceptions of EBP held by occupational therapists working in the south of England and the factors that enabled and prevented them from implementing EBP.

This research utilized qualitative and quantitative methodologies in two distinct phases. Initially, focus groups were used to explore the views and perceptions of EBP that occupational therapists working in different settings held. In the second phase, the findings from the focus groups were used to design a questionnaire to canvas the views and perceptions of a larger number of senior occupational therapists. Throughout the study, multitriangulation was used to enhance the quality and validity of the findings.

METHODS
Defining triangulation

Triangulation is a term that is commonly used in research. It was developed as a means of ensuring that research was highly creative, rigorous and systematic, in addition to enhancing its credibility and quality. It was originally introduced as a means of confirming results through the use of two or more data collection instruments and techniques to overcome the bias of single-method, single-observer or single-theory approaches (Denzin 1989).

There are two purposes of triangulation: confirmation and completeness (Shih 1998). When the aim of using triangulation is confirmation, it is expected that the results obtained through the use of two or more data collection instruments or techniques will converge. The assumption is that if similar results are obtained using different instruments or techniques then the results have greater credibility and validity. This use of triangulation is common within quantitative research.

Completeness is the second purpose of triangulation, and is more relevant to qualitative researchers. When used for completeness, different data collection instruments and techniques are used to capture a holistic view of the phenomenon being studied. The use of triangulation in this way offers depth and breadth, leading to a greater understanding of the phenomenon as each research strategy contributes a different piece of the puzzle. Thus divergent results enrich the explanations for the phenomenon.

Four types of triangulation have been identified by Denzin (1989) and critiqued by Sim & Sharp (1998). These are described in Box 10.1. It is important to realize, however, that triangulation does not have to be compartmentalized into these

Box 10.1 Four types of triangulation identified by Denzin (1989)

1. *Data triangulation* is the use of different sampling strategies and sources to compare and cross-check the consistency of information and to obtain a diverse view of the same phenomenon.
    a. *Time triangulation* refers to the collection of data at different intervals.
    b. *Space triangulation* is the collection of data on the same phenomenon in two or more settings.
    c. *Person triangulation* is the collection of information from different individuals, groups, communities, organizations or societies.
2. *Researcher triangulation* occurs when two or more researchers are involved in the analysis of the data in an attempt to compensate for single-researcher bias.
3. *Theoretical triangulation* is the use of two or more theoretical perspectives with the same data to understand how the findings are affected by different assumptions and principles.
4. *Methodological triangulation* is the use of two or more research methods or approaches in one study.
    a. *Within-method triangulation* is the use of two or more different methods within the same research paradigm (i.e. qualitative or quantitative).
    b. *Across-method triangulation* refers to the use of both qualitative and quantitative approaches in the same study.

four types. These types can be combined to gain a greater understanding of the phenomenon being studied. To meet the aims of their research, the present authors used several methods of triangulation.

Study design

Multiple triangulation was incorporated into the study design in several ways. In the first stage, triangulation was used for the purpose of completeness, and in the second stage for the purpose of confirmation.

Stage one: focus groups

Two types of triangulation were used in this stage of the research: data (more specifically space) and researcher triangulation.

In the first stage, focus groups were used as they enabled the clarification of attitudes to a particular development or experience, among a specific group – in this case, EBP among occupational therapists with at least 2 years' experience post-graduation. Focus groups encourage people to talk to one another and to ask questions, exchange anecdotes and comment on each other's experiences and points of view (Hollis et al 2002). These group processes can help people to express, consider and clarify their views, and this – in conjunction with analysis of interpersonal communication within the group – provides an insight into group norms, values and attitudes (Hollis et al 2002, Sim & Snell 1996).

In the study, the focus groups were used to tap into the views and beliefs held by senior occupational therapists about EBP. The themes and issues that emerged from the analysis of the focus groups were used as the basis for the development of the quantitative phase of the study – the postal questionnaire.

Focus group participants were recruited via letters sent to managers of occupational therapy services asking whether they could release an experienced member of staff for one morning for participation in the study. This initial letter was followed by a telephone call if the response sheet was not returned within the allocated time. Of the 28 managers contacted, 21 were able to release staff for the study.

A total of 27 senior occupational therapists attended the three focus groups. The groups were segregated along employer lines (space triangulation). The views of occupational therapists working in three different types of service (three different spaces) were sought to obtain a diverse range of opinions on which to formulate the questionnaire. Eleven attended the group for large referral hospital-based therapists, nine attended the group for small community hospital-based therapists, and seven attended the group for therapists who work primarily in the community.

Focus group protocol The focus group protocol consisted of broad questions with some prompts. The aim of these was to generate discussion between group members on the various issues, rather than to elicit answers to specific questions. The questions are listed in Box 10.2.

Box 10.2 Focus group protocol: questions and prompts

- What do you understand by the term evidence-based practice?
- In general do you think evidence-based practice is 'a good thing'?
- In an ideal world do you think occupational therapists should be carrying out evidence-based practice?
- What is the relationship between evidence-based practice and client-centred practice?
- Are you trying to use an evidence base in your day-to-day work with patients/clients?
- Is it feasible to develop more evidence-based practice in your day-to-day work? What are the sorts of things you do that could be considered evidence based?
- Do you see the professional body or special interest groups having a role to play in the development and practice of evidence-based practice?
- What sorts of things prevent you from doing more evidence-based practice?
- What sorts of things would enable you to conduct more evidence-based practice?

Focus group data collection The groups were conducted at the same venue and lasted for between one and a quarter, and one and a half hours. Before the focus groups refreshments were served, consent forms were signed, and the aims of the group and roles of the facilitator (E.J.) and observer (M.C.) were explained.

All the groups were lively and the vast majority of participants engaged with the discussion. A wide range of views and opinions was expressed, with free-flowing debate on all the topics that were introduced. The groups were all tape recorded (with the participants' permission) and fully transcribed.

Summaries of the focus groups were sent to all participants for their comments and to verify that the summary reflected a true account of the discussion. This aspect of data triangulation is an example of member checking.

Focus group data analysis During the analysis of focus group transcripts, researcher triangulation was used to enhance the reliability of the analysis and to ensure that the themes emerging from the data would be developed in a rigorous and systematic way. The verbatim transcripts of

the focus groups were independently analysed by the authors together with a third person who had extensive experience in the analysis of qualitative research data. We independently immersed ourselves in the transcripts. We tried to put aside our prior assumptions and interpretations to facilitate the possibility of reading only what the members of the focus groups were saying. This process of researchers recognizing their own thoughts and presuppositions and then attempting to suspend and bracket these when interpreting the data has been described more fully by Moustakas (1994) and Finlay (1998, 1999). Once we had exhausted our independent analysis, we met to discuss the themes that each of us had identified. Through long in-depth discussions we identified consistent themes that had emerged from the data.

On the whole, the focus group participants felt that EBP was a good thing, even though no consensus was reached on what activities constituted EBP. The participants felt there were positive benefits to doing EBP, especially in terms of improving clinical practice, raising the profile of occupational therapy and as a means of obtaining funds for equipment and continuing professional development.

There was concern, however, that EBP was not compatible with the way occupational therapists work and as a result may narrow their practice and make their interventions less creative. In addition it was felt that there were many aspects of occupational therapy intervention for which it would be difficult to research and find evidence.

The factors that prevent and enable EBP as discussed in the focus groups were related and, as such, only the enabling factors will be summarized. To enable EBP, respondents wanted:

- time built into the work schedule for EBP
- support from management
- financial support to fund continuing professional development
- more guidance from the professional body
- training in how to do and use EBP and information technology
- evidence that is reviewed and packaged ready for clinicians to implement.

Mixing methods and combining methodologies

The use of the questionnaire as the data collection tool in the second phase of this research meant that across-method triangulation was used. Across-method triangulation may be considered controversial because of the concern about combining methods from opposing research paradigms. The problem lies in the ability to integrate fully the data gathered from different methodologies (Sim & Sharp 1998). For example, data gathered from the focus groups and from the survey may differ so greatly as to prevent any meaningful combination or comparison of the data obtained by each.

The underlying reason for this problem is that the foundational philosophies and assumptions of each method are not compatible. The rationalistic paradigm assumes that reality can be measured objectively and that there is a single truth, whereas the naturalistic paradigm assumes there are multiple truths and realities cannot be measured objectively:

'A choice of data collection method entails assumptions about the nature of social life [and as such] the arbitrary combination of methods proposed by some advocates of triangulation can very easily lead the researcher into the trap of simultaneously endorsing mutually contradictory conceptualisations of the basic nature of the phenomenon under examination' (Sim & Sharp 1998, p. 28).

It can be argued that if methods from opposing paradigms generate different kinds of knowledge they should remain apart. It may be counter-argued that methods should be selected – and, where appropriate, combined – on the basis of whether this is appropriate for the research, not in terms of epistemological considerations (Connelly et al 1997). It seems that there is no right or wrong answer as to whether it is appropriate to combine methods from the two paradigms. It has been suggested, however, that there are three types of researcher: the *purist*, the *situationalist* and the *pragmatist* (Connelly et al 1997).

The *purist researcher* believes that it is not possible to mix methodologies with mutually exclusive epistemological and ontological assumptions, and tends to favour one paradigm over the other. The *situationalist researcher* uses methodologies from both paradigms but will be selective depending on

the situation. Generally, this type of researcher will use both methods in a parallel manner or in different phases, with little integration during the procedure and data analysis. Finally, the *pragmatist researcher* argues that methods can be integrated in a single study and pays little concern to the epistemological variance. This type of researcher generally advocates the use of all available techniques and views triangulation as a means of obtaining a richer, more insightful, analysis of complex data.

Each researcher must decide which philosophical orientation will inform their own approach to research. Whichever they choose, they have a responsibility to be methodical in reporting sufficient details both of their data collection and of the processes of analysis to permit others to judge the quality of the resulting product (Patton 1990). We chose to be situationalistic in the approach to our research.

Stage two: the questionnaire

Researcher triangulation was used to design the questionnaire. The authors worked together with another researcher who had experience in both questionnaire design and researching EBP. Together we initially discussed the findings that emerged from the focus group data. These themes were discussed, together with the findings that were reported in other EBP studies. The focus of these discussions was to decide the questions to be included in the postal questionnaire. The questionnaire was developed with a mixture of open, closed and Likert Scale questions. Eight versions of the questionnaire were rejected before we agreed on the rationale and precise wording of each question. The development of the covering letter was equally rigorous as it was considered essential that the letter would 'sell' the questionnaire to the respondents.

Cognitive interview testing Draft copies of the letter and questionnaire were tested using cognitive interviewing and a postal pilot with selected members of the questionnaire target group. This strategy, known as 'member checking' is one aspect of researcher triangulation.

Cognitive interviewing can be used to test survey questions in one-to-one interview settings. It is recognized as an excellent means of identifying flawed questions and should be used in conjunction with traditional piloting techniques rather than as a substitute for these (Campanelli 1997). In cognitive interviewing, respondents are encouraged to 'think aloud' as they answer the questionnaire. Campanelli (1997) suggests that cognitive interviewing can be conducted either while the respondent is completing the questionnaire or retrospectively, where respondents are interviewed, reminded of the questions and their answers, and asked to remember what they were thinking. One limitation of the concurrent method is that thinking aloud may break the natural flow of the survey questions and hence affect the answers a respondent may give to subsequent questions. A limitation of the retrospective method is that it relies on a respondent's memory.

Either method of using the 'think aloud' technique will involve the use of predetermined or spontaneous questions aimed to encourage the respondents to open up and to explore the issues that they are having with the questionnaire. This type of probing questioning is essential if the 'think aloud' technique is to be effective.

The 'think aloud' technique of cognitive interviewing appears to have several advantages. A lot of information can be gathered with relatively minimal effort and with a small number of respondents. In addition, the feedback on the questionnaire is usually in depth. Unlike pilot testing, this type of cognitive interviewing can result in more appropriate information being gathered. Furthermore, respondents can verbalize their feedback, which may be easier for many of them than writing.

The concurrent method of 'thinking aloud' was used primarily to test the draft research information letter and questionnaire as we had limited time and felt that this method would provide us with the information required. We also wanted to observe the respondents' reactions as they opened the envelope, read the information letter and completed the survey questions. We felt that by observing their responses we would be better able to probe when they found it difficult or showed signs of not understanding or of losing interest.

Two clinically experienced occupational therapists were selected to participate in the cognitive interviews. They were interviewed separately. Each interview commenced with an explanation of what was expected of the therapist and an opportunity to practise 'thinking aloud'. Following Campanelli's (1997) suggestion, each therapist was asked to try to visualize where they lived and to count the windows in the house. As they counted the windows, the therapists were encouraged to talk about what they were seeing and what they were thinking about.

After this preparation exercise, each interviewee was handed an envelope that contained the research information letter and the postal questionnaire. The therapists were asked to 'think aloud' as they opened the envelope, read the letter and answered each of the questions from the questionnaire. As the interviewees read and completed the questionnaire, prompts such as 'Tell me what you are thinking' and 'What is difficult about that question/sentence' were used to encourage the respondent to 'think aloud'. When the interviewees had completed the questionnaire, they were asked about their thoughts and feelings related to the questionnaire.

Both of the cognitive interviews were audiotaped and analysed. We then discussed the comments made by both interviewees. As a result, several changes to the wording of the information letter and the wording and design of the questionnaire were implemented. The revised letter and questionnaire were then used in the postal pilot.

Pilot questionnaire sample Fourteen pilot questionnaires were sent to four occupational therapy managers who volunteered to distribute them to members of their teams. Of these, nine were returned within the 7-day timescale – a response rate of 64%. All of the respondents completed the questionnaire correctly and made no comments suggesting changes. Therefore, no further changes were made. As no changes were made following the pilot, data from the pilot questionnaires were used in the final analysis.

Postal questionnaire sample The sample group for the postal questionnaire comprised occupational therapists who were registered to supervise students by the School of Health Professions and Rehabilitation Sciences, University of Southampton, UK. A total of 671 occupational therapists were included in this database covering the southern part of England. Occupational therapists from this database who had already been involved in the study as participants in a focus group, cognitive interview or pilot questionnaire were excluded from the sample for the postal questionnaire.

Postal questionnaire protocol The aim of the postal questionnaire was to gain detailed information from a large number of therapists about their use, views and opinions of EBP. The questionnaire was divided into four main sections. Section one asked for demographic information about each respondent. Section two was concerned with the therapists' current engagement with various EBP activities, such as reading journal articles, involvement with special interest groups, developing and implementing guidelines for practice, and maintaining continuing professional development diaries. Section three explored the therapists' views and opinions about EBP using a three-point Likert scale. It also asked therapists to state whether or not they were currently using any evidence base for their practice. The first half of section four required therapists to assess how helpful different factors would be in enabling them to develop and conduct EBP using a three-point Likert scale. In the final part of the questionnaire, there were open questions regarding factors that have prevented or enabled the therapist in conducting EBP.

Postal questionnaire data collection To achieve the maximum response rate, multiple postings were employed. The postal questionnaire, covering letter and freepost return envelope were sent to each occupational therapist in the sample and a return date was given for its return. Returned questionnaires were then logged so that non-responders could be sent another letter with a duplicate questionnaire; this procedure was then repeated, with an appropriate time lag. Thus, over a period of 2 months non-responders would have received the questionnaire three times. Questionnaires were sent to 653 occupational therapists; 500 were completed and returned, making an overall response rate of 76.5%, which is considered high for a postal survey.

Postal questionnaire data analysis Information from the closed questions on the postal questionnaire was entered into SPSSR version 8.0, and frequencies, descriptive statistics and cross-tabulations were performed. Information from the open questions was entered, verbatim, into an Access database; all the data were coded, and analysis of these codes was conducted.

SUMMARY OF RESEARCH FINDINGS

- The occupational therapists involved in this research overwhelmingly felt that EBP was a good thing. Although there were many concerns, the potential benefits to the improvement of professional practice and the development of departments were considered to be extremely beneficial.

- There was no clear definition of EBP amongst the participants. They were generally familiar with the link between research and EBP, but tended to ignore or at least downplay the value of quantitative research. They preferred to emphasize the value of clinical experience and discussion with colleagues.

- Participants considered many of the activities that they do, such as problem-solving with colleagues, attending courses, reading articles and doing presentations, as contributing to the development of an evidence base in their practice.

- Support, access to resources and personal motivation were rated as important factors that enable EBP. Support included interest and assistance from colleagues and encouragement from seniors and managers. Managers and colleagues committed to EBP appeared to be major keys to ensuring that staff use EBP. The resources that therapists found useful included access to computers and the internet, access to a medical library, and the availability of relevant articles. Personal motivation included factors such as having a personal interest in EBP, working in one's own time, having facilities at home, and having a specific reason or need to find and implement the evidence.

- Lack of time, high staff turnover, staff shortages and lack of training were rated as common preventive factors. Occupational therapists did not feel they had the time to commit to searching for, discussing and implementing the evidence when there were so many other aspects of their job that took immediate priority. Staffing problems made developing an evidence-based work ethos difficult, as did a lack of knowledge of how to implement EBP.

Overview of research

The use of multitriangulation strategies enhanced the quality of the research and the validity of the findings. While it cannot be claimed that the findings are representative of all occupational therapists working in the UK or internationally, it can be stated that the findings do reflect the views and opinions of the occupational therapists working in the southern part of England.

To move this research on and to discuss how occupational therapists can work towards developing a more evidenced-based practice, the results of this research were used as the basis for an EBP conference.

USING THE RESEARCH TO INFLUENCE PRACTICE

THE EBP CONFERENCE

A free one-day conference was held for occupational therapists who had participated in the research in some way, either through focus groups, cognitive interview testing of the questionnaire, pilot testing of the questionnaire or completing the final version of the questionnaire.

More than 100 participants attended the conference, which was run in three distinct sessions. First, there were four presentations by nurses and therapists who had research experience of EBP. The topics that were covered included the future of EBP, the role of the national body in promoting EBP, the use of qualitative research to develop EBP and, finally, how to implement a critically appraised service. This first session was to set the scene and inform participants of various issues of EBP. The second session centred on the presentation of the findings of the EBP research. Finally, the third session was a general discussion of the findings followed by small discussion groups focusing on how to apply EBP in the workplace. In the small discussion groups, participants were given two tasks to complete, as outlined in Box 10.3.

A summary of the discussions that took place at the conference is presented below. This summary is included as a way to demonstrate how EBP can become a more intrinsic part of, and prompt changes to, clinical practice.

Box 10.3 Discussion tasks for evidence-based practice conference groups

Task one: implementing changes
The research found that the following factors were considered to be the most important to enable more EBP to be conducted. Please consider how these could be implemented in your workplace:

- support
- access to resources
- time
- personal factors.

Task two: EBP activities
The following activities were identified in the focus groups and in the questionnaire as possible activities currently done by occupational therapists that could be used to develop an EBP. Choose one or more of the activities and consider how you could make it more relevant to EBP (e.g. reading journal articles in a more critical way, comparing evidence with other articles and considering/implementing changes to clinical practice rather than simply skim-reading them):

- reading journal articles
- journal club
- literature searches
- involvement with special interest groups
- attending conferences
- feeding back course information to work colleagues
- presentations
- developing and implementing guidelines for practice
- maintaining a continuing professional development diary
- using clinical experience to influence practice
- problem-solving with colleagues about clients/patients
- using objective measures to assess whether clients/patients are improving.

Recognizing qualitative research, clinical experience and client-centred practice

Participants at the conference confirmed that they were very positive about the concept of EBP. Some reservations expressed by participants centred on the fact that quantitative research – and, more specifically, randomized controlled trials – were considered to provide the best evidence. However, participants felt that, in general, this type of research was not only difficult to understand, but, more importantly, was not applicable to their practice (Egan et al 1998, Sumsion 1997).

Participants indicated a preference for qualitative styles of research as these appeared to have more relevance to occupational therapy practice. In the hierarchy of evidence, however, this type of research is rated low, and is considered to be more beneficial in generating and developing theories with less emphasis on generalizability (Bury & Jerosch-Herold 1998).

Participants were also concerned that their clinical experience was rated low in the hierarchy of evidence. It has been argued in occupational therapy and other medical literature that this should not be the case (Taylor 2000). The assumption that randomized controlled trials are the best way to evaluate the effectiveness of interventions negates the development of the reflective practitioner and consequently the influence of clinical experience. Clinical experience can be a valuable tool in the process of deciding the most appropriate intervention, especially if it has been based on reflective practice. By reflecting on experience in a structured and analytical way, new knowledge and theory can be generated through practice. It is suggested that artistry, intuition and clinical experience must complement scientific and empirical evidence, especially as it is not considered feasible to base every intervention on best evidence (Taylor 2000). This is primarily because randomized controlled trials have limited application in many interventions. These trials tend to take the average and do not consider the extremes or the individuality of each person.

The tendency towards more qualitative styles of research within occupational therapy may reflect the underlying philosophies of the profession. Occupational therapy was founded on an ethos of care, compassion and vocation, being originally practice, rather than academic, based. The move towards EBP challenges this foundation, as it appears that conflicting skills and values are required: objectivity rather than subjectivity, quantities rather than qualities, distance rather than rapport, logic rather than intuition, and dispassion rather than compassion (Hicks 1997). Qualitative research appears to be more congruent with the skills and ethos of the profession.

Participants also raised the issue of whether EBP can sit comfortably with client-centred practice. The conflict stems from the assumption that EBP further supports the concept of the practitioner being the 'expert' who determines the course of intervention, rather than the client. Client-centred practice intrinsically incorporates the concept of respect for, and partnership with, the people receiving services. As Sumsion (1997) states (p. 373):

'...[Client-centred practice] recognises the autonomy of individuals; the need for client choice in making decisions about their needs; the strength a client brings to the encounter; the benefits of the client–therapist partnership; the need to ensure that services are accessible and fit the context in which a client lives.'

An individual's life, rights and preferences must be taken into account during the decision-making process. External clinical evidence should inform but not replace clinical expertise, in which a client's rights and preferences are taken into account. Clients need to become active participants in their care. The clinician may be able to decide what evidence applies to the client but then has to develop skills to present this evidence in an objective and informative way. This enables the client to be actively involved in the decision-making process, which has involved the use of evidence-based interventions. When used in this way, client-centred practice and evidence-based practice can be compatible.

Working together to foster EBP within departments

When developing an EBP ethos, participants considered it essential for the majority of staff in a department to be interested in EBP, particularly because it was believed that a commitment to EBP was time consuming and continual. An ethos of EBP needed to be fostered within the department, and the importance of EBP needed to be continually reinforced. Managers needed to ensure that the issue of EBP came up in staff appraisals and was a focus at staff meetings. Staff searching for research evidence need to be able to do so without feeling that they are not fulfilling their work duties by having time out from working with clients.

Support for EBP is essential for another reason. It became clear throughout the research and during the conference that occupational therapists generally considered EBP an individual responsibility. Hence therapists talked a lot about having time dedicated to finding evidence to support their own practice. EBP was looked at as something that could be slotted into the working week of each therapist if they had dedicated time in which to do it. This indicated that therapists did not necessarily see EBP as being intrinsic to their everyday practice, and was based on the assumption that each person was responsible for finding their own evidence.

It became evident during the discussion at the conference that working within a department that had an ethos of EBP also meant working together to find and implement the evidence. This meant that the development of EBP was seen as a joint responsibility. Through discussion and negotiation, the therapists in various teams need to identify their priorities for EBP. These priorities should then be worked through in a logical manner with tasks assigned to various team members so that each priority is manageable and becomes a team project.

Conroy (1997) provides an example of this when coordinating a project in which nine paediatric occupational therapists were involved in searching for evidence of efficacy in their clinical practice. The therapists divided themselves into three groups related to their main area of work: those working with children who primarily had a physical impairment, those working with children who primarily had emotional and behavioural impairments, and those working with children

who had special needs but were attending mainstream schools. Each group of therapists had to agree on a topic that they wanted to investigate and then devise a statement that would indicate the aim of the investigation. With the assistance of an experienced researcher, each group searched for articles related to the topic and statement. The articles were distributed between the group members and were critiqued according to an agreed format. The articles were discussed by therapists at regular meetings. Following on from these discussions, the therapists wrote a summary of the investigation findings and the relevance of these findings to clinical practice. Consideration was also given to future topics to be investigated.

Conroy's (1997) article identifies a process that teams can use to find the evidence for their practice. This process involves teamwork rather than individual effort. Through teamwork, the finding and sorting of evidence is not only a quicker process but also a means of ensuring support within a department.

Using journal clubs to discuss the evidence

The process put forward by Conroy (1997) also points to the need for departments to agree on their priorities and to be committed to achieving them if the development of practice based on evidence is to become a reality. This is also the case when running a journal club. A journal club is made up of a group of therapists who meet regularly (the frequency depends on what is being investigated) to review and discuss articles relevant to their practice (Taylor 2000). Effective journal clubs provide a team approach to investigating and discussing topics of interest, and alleviate some of the onus on individuals being responsible for their own development of EBP (Dingle & Hooper 2000). Guidelines for establishing a journal club are put forward by Taylor (2000), while Dingle & Hooper (2000) describe the experience of establishing one. Journal clubs were felt by the conference group to be an effective means to maintain staff's professional development. To be effective, support and time needs to be given to running the journal club and to enabling staff to search for and read relevant articles. Furthermore, the club should focus on one topic at a time rather than every member bringing in a different article. Such journal clubs facilitate collaborative and effective review, discussion and critiquing of articles relevant to occupational therapy practice.

Learning the skills necessary to develop EBP

A major factor in the development of EBP was staff perceptions that they lacked the skills necessary to do EBP. Therapists need to feel a level of competence if they are to become involved in EBP. Two main aspects of this perception of competence were raised. First, many therapists, particularly those who have not recently graduated, felt that they lacked the computer skills required to search for research evidence. Second, many therapists believed that they did not have the skills necessary to appraise research articles critically; often this referred to not understanding the research component of an article.

Participants suggested that recently graduated staff who had learnt research skills in their undergraduate training could assist other staff members in developing the skills they felt they lacked. Working together as a team means that tasks can also be shared to ensure that each therapist's skills can be used effectively. For example, one therapist may be assigned to do the computer searches but all therapists can be involved in deciding the topic, and suggesting the statement and keywords to be used when searching.

Therapists who feel they do not have the skills for critically appraising the literature can still read the articles and provide their comments, but learn from others about the appropriateness of the methodology and research process. Therapists with an understanding of research can comment on those aspects, while staff with clinical experience can comment on the relevance of the findings to practice.

In addition to postgraduate courses, there are many books, articles and websites that can be used to assist people in developing skills to enable them to search for and appraise the evidence.

Attending courses

Participants stated that attending courses is an effective way of learning new practical skills, and this is probably the most common means by which therapists update their skills. Turner & Whitfield (1997) found that therapists were more likely to implement what they had learnt from a course compared with what they had read in an article. As courses have this positive effect, it is important for therapists to be discerning about which ones they attend. Courses need to be selected on the basis of whether there is a strong evidence base or, if this is not the case, on whether there is time to discuss the implications of the findings in the light of the lack of evidence. Course organizers need to be questioned about the evidence base supporting what they teach.

Resources

Lack of access to appropriate resources was a major issue for many participants. Predominantly, the resources that therapists wanted access to were the internet and facilities for searching journal databases. This was not an easy issue to solve as it depended on whether these resources were available locally, whether therapists had access to these resources at home, or whether there were financial reserves to pay for these resources. Some therapists will have access to local resources such as medical libraries; however, many work a considerable distance from such services and hence this is not convenient. If resources are not conveniently located, therapists are less likely to use them. There is no easy solution to this issue, but departments cannot ignore it. There needs to be some discussion on how best to access resources to facilitate EBP.

Working in small teams

Working in a small team was considered to be a disadvantage as there was either no one, or only a very small number of other staff, with whom to share the complex tasks of developing EBP. No solutions on how to deal with this issue were suggested by the participants and it is possible that the solution for each small team will be different, depending on their circumstances. It was suggested that solo therapists and small groups might be able to join up with others in the same situation or could look at becoming part of a multidisciplinary group, although it was recognized that for therapists working in this type of setting this was very difficult.

SUMMARY

This chapter was separated into two distinct but connected sections. The first section detailed the methodology that was used in the research investigating occupational therapists' views and perceptions of EBP. The detailed methodology was provided to enable readers to understand the complexity of the research process and how qualitative and quantitative methods can be combined to enhance the validity and reliability of research.

The second section summarized the discussions of a group of occupational therapists who attended a one-day conference centred on the findings of the research conducted by the two authors. There were two main reasons for including this section. First, it was to demonstrate how the findings of research can be used as a basis for discussion on how to apply research findings to practice. Second, it was considered that the issues raised in the discussions would have relevance to other occupational therapists and might stimulate innovative ways in which therapists could work in a more evidence-based way. The next stage is to present and share examples of good practice for others to learn from. This is a challenge for all practising occupational therapists.

REFERENCES

Barnard S, Wiles R 2001 Evidence-based physiotherapy: physiotherapists' attitudes and experiences in the Wessex area. Physiotherapy 87(3):115–124

Bury T, Jerosch-Herold C 1998 Reading and critical appraisal of the literature. In: T Bury, J Mead (eds) Evidence-based healthcare: a practical guide for therapists. Butterworth-Heinemann, Oxford; pp. 136–161

Campanelli P 1997 Testing survey questions: new directions in cognitive interviewing. Bulletin de Methodologie Sociologie 55:5–17

Closs SJ, Lewin B 1998 Perceived barriers to research utilisation: a survey of four therapies. British Journal of Therapy and Rehabilitation 5(3):151–155

Connelly L, Bott M, Hoffart N, Taunton R 1997 Methodological triangulation in a study of nurse retention. Nursing Research 45(5):299–302

Conroy MC 1997 'Why are you doing that?' A project to look for evidence of efficacy within occupational therapy. British Journal of Occupational Therapy 60(11):487–490

Cusick A, McCluskey A 2000 Becoming an evidence-based practitioner through professional development. Australian Occupational Therapy Journal 47:159–170

Denzin N 1989 The research act: a theoretical introduction to sociological methods. 3rd edn. McGraw Hill, New York

Dingle J, Hooper L 2000 Establishing a journal club in an occupational therapy service: one service's experience. British Journal of Occupational Therapy 63(11):554–556

Dubouloz C, Egan M, Vallerand J, von Zweck C 1999 Occupational therapists' perceptions of evidence-based practice. American Journal of Occupational Therapy 53(4):445–453

Egan M, Dubouloz C, von Zweck C, Vallerand J 1998 The client-centred evidence-based practice of occupational therapy. Canadian Journal of Occupational Therapy 63(3):136–143

Finlay L 1998 Reflexivity: an essential component for all research. British Journal of Occupational Therapy 61(10):453–456

Finlay L 1999 Applying phenomenology in research: problems, principles and practice. British Journal of Occupational Therapy 62(7):299–306

Hicks C 1997 The dilemma of incorporating research into clinical practice. British Journal of Nursing 6(9):511–515

Hollis V, Openshaw S, Goble R 2002 Conducting focus groups: purpose and practicalities. British Journal of Occupational Therapy 65(1):2–8

Moustakas C 1994 Phenomenological research methods. Sage, Thousand Oaks, CA

Patton M 1990 Qualitative evaluation and research methods. 2nd edn. Sage, Newbury Park, CA

Pringle E 1999 EBP: is it for me? Therapy Weekly 10 June:12

Shih F 1998 Triangulation in nursing research: issues of conceptual clarity and purpose. Journal of Advanced Nursing 28(3):631–641

Sim J, Sharp K 1998 A critical appraisal of the role of triangulation in nursing research. International Journal of Nursing Studies 35:23–31

Sim J, Snell J 1996 Focus groups in physiotherapy evaluation and research. Physiotherapy 82(3):189–198

Sumsion T 1997 Client-centred implications of evidence-based practice. Physiotherapy 83(7):373–374

Taylor MC 2000 Evidence-based practice for occupational therapists. Blackwell Science, Oxford

Turner P, Whitfield T 1997 Physiotherapists' use of evidence-based practice: a cross-national study. Physiotherapy Research International 2(1):17–29

Upton D 1999 Clinical effectiveness and EBP 2: attitudes of health care professionals. British Journal of Therapy and Rehabilitation 6(1):26–30

FURTHER READING

Curtin M, Jaramazovic E 2001 Occupational therapists' views and perceptions of evidence-based practice. British Journal of Occupational Therapy 64(5):214–222

Denzin N, Lincoln Y (eds) 2000 Handbook of qualitative research. 2nd edn. Sage, Thousand Oaks, CA

11

Using qualitative evidence as a basis for evidence-based practice

Karen Whalley Hammell

OVERVIEW

This final chapter builds on the themes of client-centred philosophy and participatory research that have been explored in the previous chapters, examining whether client-centred practice has a supportive evidence base and whether evidence exists to demonstrate that current imperatives for consumer involvement in research have been met by the rehabilitation professions. Drawing together published research literature, Karen Whalley Hammell explores how qualitative evidence is being used to inform theory, education and practice, to evaluate outcomes and assess quality of life, and to evaluate and plan service delivery. This exploration introduces methods of qualitative research not yet addressed in this book: institutional ethnography, the Delphi technique and the nominal group technique. Discussion of the place and role of qualitative evidence in systematic reviews demands consideration of the quality and rigour of qualitative inquiry; thus the chapter suggests a framework of guidelines for evaluating qualitative research. Finally, the chapter further explores the potential for mixing the methods of qualitative and quantitative research to address the complex issues presented to rehabilitation therapists. Overall, the intent of this chapter is to provide qualitative research evidence to demonstrate the potential for informing practice through relevant and useful qualitative research.

INTRODUCTION

This chapter builds on the preceding chapters in illustrating some of the many ways in which the evidence derived from qualitative research can be used to inform practice. Methods of qualitative research not previously addressed in this book will be sketched and their potential contributions to evidence-based practice outlined (i.e. institutional ethnography, Delphi technique, nominal group technique, systematic reviews). The chapter briefly reviews some suggested guidelines with which to evaluate the rigour of reported qualitative research (and hence its authority to inform evidence-based practice) and examines the potential and possibilities for mixing the methods of qualitative research with those of quantitative research.

CLIENT-CENTRED PHILOSOPHY

Chapter 1 alluded to innovations in government policies that require healthcare services to be responsive to the needs of users, and acknowledgement by the rehabilitation professions that consumers must be involved both in designing models of service delivery and in identifying modes of intervention that best meet their needs. While client-centred practice has long been advocated by occupational therapists (e.g. Canadian Association of Occupational Therapists 1983), and more recently by physical therapists (e.g. MacDonald et al 2001), it is evident that this has become a required – rather than an optional – modus operandi (Hammell 2003).

Many of the contributors to this book have demonstrated their commitment to client-centred practices by involving clients in every dimension of the research process and by striving to ensure that professional theories, modes of practice and models of service delivery are informed by client perspectives. But does client-centred practice have a supportive evidence base?

Client-centred practice: an evidence-based mode of practice

Law (1998a) reviewed the research literature from diverse healthcare disciplines to determine whether client-centred practice could be considered an effective means of service delivery. She concluded from this review that research evidence supports the premise that client-centred practice leads to improved client satisfaction and outcomes. Further, she reported that research evidence demonstrates that: 'Time and resources are maximized because therapy focuses on the issues which are most important to the person and his or her family' (Law 1998b, p. xv). Similar findings have been reported by other researchers (e.g. Fischer et al 1999). Because research evidence supports client-centred service delivery, it can therefore be claimed that client-centred practice is an evidence-based mode of practice.

Consumer involvement in research: principles

So far, the chapters in this book have highlighted the contemporary imperative for the inclusion of clients' voices in decisions pertaining to their own care, and has referred to research evidence that supports this client-centred mode of practice.

Critics contend, however, that if therapists espouse client-centred practice it follows that client involvement must extend to the research undertaken to inform service delivery (Hammell 2001). In Canada, the USA and Australia, for example, legislated mandates require the inclusion of clients in the process of evaluating health care and health promotion programmes (Clark et al 1993, Twible 1992).

Undertaking research that is designed to inform client-centred practice and that is ethically consistent with the espousal of client-centred ideals demands a conscious realignment of power and a deliberate effort to include clients as collaborators at every stage of the research process, from the initial identification of an issue for study through data collection and analysis to the dissemination of findings (Hammell 2001). If therapists define their own research agendas and use research methods that exclude the perspectives and voices of their clients, then any resulting 'evidence' will inevitably be framed within parameters determined by therapists' values, assumptions, priorities and objectives, and will be of questionable relevance as a basis for practice (Hammell 2001). Indeed, disability theorists contend that 'disabled people have come to see research ... as irrelevant to their needs' (Oliver 1996, p. 141).

Recognizing the necessity for client-centred practice to match client-centred rhetoric, the 2001 College of Occupational Therapists' Research and Development Strategic Vision and Action Plan in the UK (Ilott & White 2001) stated clearly, 'researchers are ... expected to act collaboratively, involving consumers at all levels and stages of the research process' (p. 270), and 'Research and evidence-based practice is expected to incorporate a user perspective; this means involving consumers and carers throughout the research process and as partners in quality-enhancement initiatives' (p. 275). Theoretically, therefore, there is a pressing imperative for consumer involvement in research – but has this been fully translated into practice?

Consumer involvement in research: practice

Although there are clear political, ethical and social imperatives for involving consumers in the entire research process, a review of the literature reveals that few occupational or physical therapists have sought to translate client-centred theory into practice by working in collaboration with clients or consumer groups. 'Many disabled people are dissatisfied with ... the process of research that provides the knowledge base for professional practice' (Thomas & Parry 1996, p. 6). Few researchers have been prepared to relinquish power and strive for participatory modes of research. Indeed, it is ironic that, while therapists have contributed their own definitions of client-centred practice (e.g. Sumsion 1999), few researchers have sought to explore the meaning of client-centred practice to clients. Deborah Corring's chapter in this book (Ch. 6) describes one of the few attempts to provide client-centred input to client-centred philosophy. Further, the chapters by Karen Rebeiro (Ch. 8), Chris Carpenter (Ch. 5) and Mary Law (Ch. 4) are exemplars of a participatory approach to research. These authors demonstrate how the skills and knowledge of researchers can be blended with the experience and knowledge of clients and consumer groups to produce evidence that is relevant and useful, and thus provide a credible basis on which to ground subsequent client-centred practice (Law), theory (Law) and service delivery, policy and programme planning (Carpenter, Law, Rebeiro).

USING QUALITATIVE EVIDENCE

Chapter 1 alluded to the preoccupation with quantitative research among the original proponents of evidence-based practice. However, more recent recognition of the value of qualitative research to a more complete and nuanced understanding of the complex issues involved in health and health care has encouraged increased attention to the use of qualitative evidence (Miller & Crabtree 2000, Pope & Mays 2000).

The examples described in the previous chapters construct both a rationale for, and examples of, how qualitative evidence can contribute to the development of theory, practice and service delivery. This section builds upon these chapters by drawing on a sample of published reports to demonstrate further how qualitative evidence can provide a relevant evidence base with which to inform theory and practice.

Using qualitative evidence to inform theory

Researchers who have examined current therapy practice have reported that approaches to intervention frequently appear to be devoid of a theoretical basis, and that when therapists do lay claim to a governing theory this theory, itself, is found to be devoid of a supporting evidence base (e.g. Davidson & Waters 2000, Walker et al 2000). Clearly, if theory informs practice (as it should), then research evidence must inform theory.

Data derived from qualitative research can be used to reaffirm, revise or expand particular theoretical frameworks, to expose limits to current theories and to identify previously unrecognized relationships among elements of a phenomenon (Hammell & Carpenter 2000, Hammell 2001).

In particular, qualitative research is valuable in enabling the incorporation of different perspectives from people who have different cultural and social positions. Variables that contribute to personal and cultural differences include, but are not limited to: professional status and education, gender, 'race', ethnicity, age, social class, sexual orientation, (dis)ability, religion, income and language (Hammell 2001). Although occupational and physical therapists tend to reflect homogeneity on many of these variables, their clients are likely to be more diverse and thus unlikely to share their therapists' value systems. Alcoff (1991, p. 7) observed: 'we are authorized by virtue of our academic positions to develop theories that express and encompass the ideas, needs, and goals of others. However, we must begin to ask ourselves whether this is a legitimate authority'. The chapters by Melinda Suto (Ch. 3) and Karen Whalley Hammell (Ch. 2) describe two attempts to enable a diversity of views to penetrate theory and to critique those perspectives derived from the particular (i.e. not universal) viewpoints of occupational therapy clinicians and academics.

Using qualitative evidence to evaluate outcomes

One of the hallmarks of a client-centred approach to practice is the involvement of clients in all aspects of intervention, including evaluation of outcomes (Clark et al 1993). A client-centred orientation requires that outcome assessments reflect the values, priorities and goals of the client rather than those of therapists – assessing outcomes that 'matter'. Considerable evidence demonstrates that clients do not share the same priorities, preoccupations or perceptions of problems as their healthcare providers (e.g. Clark et al 1993); thus a 'clinically significant' outcome may be significant only to a clinician (Ray & Mayan 2001). It has, therefore, been queried whether the purpose of judging 'successful' outcomes by measuring those outcomes prioritized by therapists is simply a means to justify and validate customary rehabilitation practice (Eisenberg & Saltz 1991).

While outcome assessments have traditionally focused on functional achievements, these constitute superficial outcome indicators, at best. Clinicians would doubtless support the observation that while 'some functionally independent patients are happy, productive and socially active. Others are not' (Woolsey 1985, p. 119). Assessment of physical function is an insufficient gauge of the usefulness or value of rehabilitation services to clients' lives (Hammell 2003).

It should be self-evident that the most important question in evaluating outcomes is: 'What outcomes are important to clients?'. Needham & Oliver (1998) attach further requirements:

- *How* can outcomes be assessed such that they reflect clients' priorities?
- From the clients' perspective, what are the most appropriate times for assessing outcomes (i.e. *when* do clients think that outcomes should be assessed?).

The incorporation of clients' priorities and perspectives requires the use of qualitative forms of assessment.

Acknowledging the need to assess outcomes that are appropriate to clients' self-assessed needs and relevant to their lives, therapists have developed assessment tools that are specifically designed to reflect clients' perspectives. In 1990, a group of Canadian occupational therapists developed the Canadian Occupational Performance Measure (Law et al 1998), which is a client-centred outcome measure used with diverse client groups (Bodiam 1999). Similarly, physical therapists in Canada have developed the Patient-Specific Functional Scale (Stratford et al 1995) to assess ability and disability in activities that are important to the individual (Westaway et al 1998). Noting the discrepancies between physicians' and patients' perspectives, medical researchers are advocating assessment of the patient's view of health status changes in both clinical practice and clinical trials. This reflects a recognition of the need to produce a greater depth of understanding about perceptions of outcomes and their importance and meaning in clients' lives (Fischer et al 1999).

Using qualitative evidence to assess quality of life

The quality of life of disabled people is often said to have been 'measured' using tools devised by researchers. This reflects an assumption that researchers can be objective and value-free, and thus design research instruments that are universally applicable (Hammell 2002). Research has demonstrated, however, that the quality of a life can be assessed only by the person whose life it is, based on their own values and priorities (e.g. Gill & Feinstein 1994). Thus Dale (1995) contends that any claims by health professionals to have measured the quality of life experienced by a patient, using current tools, are unsubstantiated.

Recognizing that researchers, clinicians and clients may have different definitions of quality of life, and of the factors deemed to contribute to the experience of a life worth living, occupational therapy researchers undertook a qualitative study to explore the perspectives of people with schizophrenia regarding the meaning of quality of life and factors perceived to be important to quality of life (Laliberte-Rudman et al 2000). Although their findings supported the importance of factors usually included in existing quality of life assessments, they also indicated the need to look at new dimensions of factors that are commonly included, in addition to including other factors that are not generally included. The researchers planned to use their qualitative evidence to develop a quality of life assessment *for* people with schizophrenia that is based on the perspectives and priorities *of* people with schizophrenia, thereby assuring the relevance and usefulness of future assessment.

Using qualitative evidence in education

Qualitative research has been used to generate evidence with which to ensure the relevance of the educational experience for occupational therapy students. Responding to the need to enable future occupational therapists to practise competently in multicultural societies, qualitative research was undertaken to explore how students developed the knowledge and skills to work with people from different social and cultural backgrounds (Whiteford & Wilcock 2000). In addition to identifying curriculum and teaching/learning processes that enhance the development of intercultural competence, the data that emerged from the study also highlighted important issues concerning the ways in which occupation and independence are conceptualized across cultures. This study therefore demonstrates the potential for using qualitative evidence to inform both the content and process of educational programmes. The research reported on by Gwyer and colleagues in Chapter 9 illustrates efforts to contribute qualitative evidence to the education of physical therapy students.

Using qualitative evidence in clinical practice

Physical therapy theory acknowledges the importance of social and cultural contexts to understanding movement (Cott et al 1995) and multiple dimensions of health (Jorgensen 2000). In an effort to determine whether theory is translated into practice, Jorgensen (2000) undertook a qualitative research project to discover what physical therapists knew about the social and cultural lives of clients who had total hip arthroplasty and how such information served to inform clinical practice. Jorgensen's findings supported the premise that a theory–practice gap exists in the physical therapy profession, revealing a mechanical view of the body and a perception of the role of the physical therapist as being that of teaching clients a standard treatment regimen rather than attempting to tailor interventions to meet their individual needs. The research findings were used to highlight the need for physical therapy assessment tools that would facilitate the identification and inclusion of clients' attitudes and values into physical therapy practice. Candice Schachter and colleagues describe in Chapter 7 how they developed principles of sensitive physical therapy practice from qualitative research that actively sought clients' input and strove to understand clients' perspectives. This study, again, facilitated the identification and inclusion of clients' attitudes and values into physical therapy practice.

Using qualitative evidence in evaluating and planning service delivery

Clark et al (1993) proposed that a client-centred approach to service delivery, by definition, will involve clients in all aspects of intervention, including programme evaluation, and that this collaboration should form the basis for planning occupational therapy services. It has been noted that: 'several studies of client involvement in service evaluation have demonstrated that clients are capable of determining what services they find most satisfying, and that *such involvement can lead to better health outcomes*' (Corring 1999, p. 8; emphasis added). These findings suggest that the opportunity for clients to participate in service evaluation may be inherently therapeutic.

Stephenson & Wiles (2000) described a qualitative study designed to explore perceptions of a home-delivered therapy service among people with stroke. Their findings demonstrated that assumptions about the advantages and disadvantages of community-based rehabilitation services made by service providers are not necessarily shared by the users of these services. The study further highlighted possible factors that might enhance clients' outcomes and their degree of satisfaction with this mode of service delivery. This study of clients' perspectives provided substantive evidence with which to make services more appropriate and relevant to clients' needs.

In Chapter 8, Karen Rebeiro alluded to the tendency for people with severe, persistent mental illnesses to experience continual readmissions to hospital. Recognizing this 'revolving-door problem' – and the disruption to the lives of patients it represented – Davidson et al (1997) engaged in participatory research with individuals diagnosed with severe mental illness that used qualitative methods to explore clients' perspectives of the precipitants and reasons for 'recidivism' and to identify possible alternatives. They demonstrated that service delivery can be effective only if it is addressing the problems perceived by service users and grounded in their experiences and perspectives. These findings provided the basis for a new approach to intervention that has helped the clients to establish more satisfying lives in the community. Davidson and colleagues recognized the limitations of their own definition of the 'problem' of recidivism, which failed to address the social and material environment to which patients returned following discharge, and which overlooked the reality that people might view a return to hospital as a legitimate alternative to life on the streets.

The clear similarities between the findings of Davidson et al (1997) and those reported in Chapter 8 by Karen Rebeiro provide corroborating evidence for the findings of both studies and demonstrate the credibility of informing service delivery with qualitative data.

Recognizing that people do not live in vacuums but in complex social worlds, qualitative methods contextualize research by enabling consideration of environmental factors that affect people's lives. However, because therapists also act within complex social worlds, research methods are required to enable these contexts to be exposed and explored.

Institutional ethnography: in theory

Therapists frequently complain about the 'systems' in which they work and the ways in which these systems subvert or thwart their efforts to practise in a client-centred manner. Canadian sociologist, Dorothy Smith (1990) developed *institutional ethnography* as a theory and qualitative method for exploring the social, political and economic processes that organize and determine everyday activities. Smith aimed to reveal how policies, procedures, statistics and other forms of documentation are interconnected and related to a ruling apparatus. Thus, institutional ethnography is concerned with explicating 'the processes through which power is routinely organized' and how 'micro, everyday experiences are interconnected with macro, systemic processes in ways that routinely perpetuate inequalities in power' (Townsend 1996, p. 181). Drawing upon Smith's work, an occupational therapist, Elizabeth Townsend (1996) observed: 'In essence, modern power is exerted through the documentary processes used to describe, categorize, define, direct, visually represent, or otherwise coordinate and control the everyday world' (p. 188).

Townsend (1996) delineated the three analytical processes employed in an institutional ethnography:

- Data analysis aimed at describing everyday practice, as revealed through participant observation, interviews and document review.
- Analysis demonstrating connections between everyday practices (e.g. policies, methods of collecting information, requisite categories of information, workload measurement systems) and the organizational processes used to coordinate and govern that practice in a particular institution.
- Analysis showing how knowledge is ideologically organized around particular, prevailing ideas. Here, for example, an analysis might ask: why are time-use, funding, caseload data and reporting techniques organized as they are? The analysis might reveal that categories of required documentation exclude dimensions pertaining to client-centred enablement of occupational performance or of functional movement, focusing instead on diagnostic categories or treatment units that reflect the more powerful ideology and dominance of medicine, thereby rendering occupational and physical therapists' work invisible. When physical therapists and occupational therapists record outcomes pertaining to range of motion and muscle strength (for example) rather than functional movements and occupations – that is, the *consequences* of range and strength for everyday lives and their congruence with clients' goals

and roles – they collude in the subordination of their own profession's values and actively obscure the importance of their work.

Institutional ethnography: in practice

Townsend (1996) used Smith's methods to show how particular organizational contexts shaped community-based occupational therapy programmes for people with mental illnesses in Atlantic Canada. Her study revealed how occupational therapists' aspirations to encourage engagement in occupations and enable the empowerment of people with mental illnesses were subverted by specific organizational processes. Moreover, she demonstrated that the therapists perpetuated their subjugation each time they participated in processes of documentation that reflected organizational, rather than occupational therapy, ideologies. Thus, occupational therapists were not victims of the inequitable systems in which they worked, but active collaborators.

Research that has sought clients' perspectives of rehabilitation demonstrates that this process is frequently experienced as being irrelevant to clients' lives, inappropriate to their roles, incongruent with their goals and focused on the implementation of standard treatment regimens rather than upon client-centred practice (e.g. Abberley 1995, Jorgensen 2000). Using institutional ethnography to generate qualitative evidence of organizational practices and their ideological impact might reveal *why* it is apparently so difficult to translate client-centred philosophy into client-centred practice, thereby creating the basis and possibility for change.

QUALITATIVE ASSESSMENT OF EVIDENCE: INTRODUCING THE DELPHI TECHNIQUE AND THE NOMINAL GROUP TECHNIQUE

Sometimes sufficient, conclusive evidence exists to inform practice, but more frequently a lack of evidence or contradictory evidence results in uncertainties and consequent inconsistencies in practice. In such circumstances consensus methods may be used to determine the extent of agreement, permitting a qualitative assessment of evidence (Jones & Hunter 2000).

Sackett et al's (2000) hierarchy of evidence (see Table 1.1) recognizes 'expert' opinion as one form of evidence upon which practice might legitimately be based (in the absence of conclusive research evidence). The term *expert* is a problematic one for therapists, implying superiority of certain sorts of knowledge (notably privileging the therapist's knowledge rather than the client's). Further, it is rarely clear upon what basis 'expertise' might legitimately be claimed: whether, for example, this is on the basis of published peer-reviewed research, attainment of a higher degree, the esteem of one's peers, or from a perception that competence somehow accrues with 'patient miles' – the number of patients treated over many years (Richardson 1999, Sumsion 1998). (The latter proposition is particularly problematic in light of early research suggesting that misperceptions of clients' problems by rehabilitation staff may actually worsen with the length of clinical experience; e.g. Bodenhamer et al 1983, Ernst 1987.) The definition of 'expert' needs to be broadened to acknowledge the experiences and knowledges of people who have different positions and perspectives based on their experiences as consumers of health care and as experts concerning their own problems and needs.

The following two sections outline two qualitative research methods that have been used successfully by physical therapists and occupational therapists to generate a consensus with which to inform subsequent research, education, theory or practice: the Delphi technique and the nominal group technique.

Both of these techniques require a measurement of the degree to which each participant agrees with an issue or statement under consideration and also the degree to which participants agree with one another. Jones & Hunter (2000) provide guidelines concerning suitable statistical procedures for these purposes.

Notably, the achievement of a consensus does not mean that a 'correct' answer has been identified: 'there is the danger of deriving collective ignorance rather than wisdom' (Jones & Hunter 2000, p. 45). Rather than viewing the results of these methods as reliable and authoritative, it is suggested that 'they should be regarded more as methods for structuring group communication on a question, than as a means for providing definitive answers' (Jones & Hunter 2000, p. 48).

Using qualitative evidence to identify research priorities: the Delphi technique

The Delphi technique is a method of qualitative research that is used to achieve a consensus and is explored in detail by Jones & Hunter (2000) and Sumsion (1998). It is used most appropriately where little evidence exists and opinions are being sought (Jones & Hunter 2000). This research method comprises a series of rounds of questionnaires (usually three or four) completed by the same group of people, such that each round builds on the results of the previous one.

In the first round, relevant individuals are invited to provide their opinions on specific issues, based on their knowledge and experience (Jones & Hunter 2000). This round comprises open-ended questions to which the participants respond. These opinions are grouped together by the researchers under headings and statements, and then circulated to every member of the group. This allows each person to see how others have responded, to identify whether pertinent information appears to have been omitted, and to review or revise their own positions. In the second round, the participants rank their degree of agreement with the various statements, and these rankings, in turn, are compiled and consolidated and returned to the group members. In the third round, the participants receive a third questionnaire and are again asked to rank their agreement with each statement. If an acceptable degree of consensus has been achieved, the process may be terminated and the results shared with the participants. If not, the third round is repeated (Jones & Hunter 2000). In the final report, the degree of consensus should be included, as a percentage (for example, 60% or 75% agreement) (Sumsion 1998).

Sumsion (1998) observed that, while the first stage of this research method had traditionally been used to generate ideas, some support exists for saving time by presenting pre-existing information (derived from the literature) for ranking or response. This would appear to be problematic, in that this constitutes limited or forced choices and precludes consideration of issues or perspectives not previously identified in the existing literature, thus relying upon 'thinking as usual'. Potential for bias exists when categories deemed worthy of consideration are predetermined by the researcher. Further, on those occasions when a participant group has been selected on the basis of professional 'expertise', a familiarity with the relevant literature could reasonably be expected as an essential component of competence.

The Delphi technique is an inexpensive way to gather information and opinions from a specific group of people who have valuable knowledge and experience to contribute. Participants can be drawn from different countries, using electronic communication, if this is congruent with the nature of the topic. The method has the benefit of enabling participants to reflect on both the issues and their responses between the various rounds, and of gleaning opinions on a wide variety of issues or problems. The number of participants varies widely, dependent upon the topic under investigation and the resources available for consolidating and distributing the questionnaires.

Clearly, the choice of participants is crucial to the plausibility and credibility of the outcomes achieved. Recourse to people who share a certain perspective (by virtue of shared educational experiences or social position, for example) will easily produce a consensus, but one that contributes only a partial insight. One of the strengths of this survey method, however, is the elimination of the effects of group dynamics and the anonymity of the participants. Sumsion (1998, p. 154) astutely observed: 'The advantages and disadvantages of this technique must be weighed against the objectives of the proposed research and the advantages and disadvantages of all other available methodologies'.

The Delphi technique has been used widely in healthcare research and is viewed as a particularly useful tool for those in management or research who wish to achieve consensus on a given issue (Sumsion 1998). The technique has been used,

for example, to determine the learning needs of physical therapy and occupational therapy staff (Barclay-Goddard & Strock 2001).

Application of the Delphi technique

The Delphi technique has been used successfully as a method of generating evidence with which to establish research priorities for physical therapists. Responding to clinicians' frustration that little published research appeared relevant to clinical practice, Miles-Tapping et al (1990) involved all physical therapists, including those in management, at a large teaching hospital in Canada in a Delphi research project that enabled consensus to be reached on priorities for clinical research. Similar research was undertaken by Walker (1994) in the UK. In this instance, two concurrent studies included physical therapists who had research experience and a second group of physical therapists who were recent graduates with little or no research experience. Substantial agreement between the two groups suggested similar concerns about the areas of research that required prompt attention within the physical therapy profession. Similarities could also be discerned between Walker's (1994) study in the UK and Miles-Tapping et al's (1990) study, published 4 years earlier in Canada. These findings suggest that the Delphi technique is a useful means of ensuring that research energies and funding are targeted towards exploring those issues that are clinically relevant – a base on which to develop evidence to inform practice. From a client-centred perspective, it would be valuable to undertake similar research with defined diagnostic groups, exploring, for example, the research priorities of people with stroke who have undergone rehabilitation programmes including occupational and physical therapy.

The nominal group technique

The nominal group technique uses a structured meeting to gather information about an issue from a group of people who have particular knowledge or experience of a given issue (usually about 9 to 12 people) (Jones & Hunter 2000). This technique is considered especially appropriate when the opinions of 'experts' are being sought *and* a body of relevant evidence exists that can be incorporated into the decision-making process (Jones & Hunter 2000).

The technique comprises two rounds in which participants rate, discuss and re-rate a series of items or questions. The meetings are facilitated by someone who is deemed to have credibility in relation to the topic (Jones & Hunter 2000). The nominal group process follows a specific structure. Initially, the participants are asked to write down their answers to a given question. Each participant contributes one idea or opinion to the facilitator, until every idea has been listed. The facilitator lists these on a board. The participants decide how similar ideas might be grouped together through a process of clarification and evaluation, and then each participant privately ranks each contribution in order of perceived importance. Once these rankings have been tabulated, presented to the group and discussed, they are re-ranked by each participant. Overall rankings are tabulated and the results presented to the group (Jones & Hunter 2000, Twible 1992). In comparison with other forms of group meeting, it has been suggested that the nominal group technique 'generates a greater flow of ideas, encourages fuller participation of all involved, allows decision making to be completed within the time allocated, and encourages participant satisfaction with the three preceding accomplishments' (Twible 1992, p. 14). This method has been used to attain a consensus of opinion on issues such as the appropriateness of specific clinical interventions, fostering discussion focused on a single issue (Jones & Hunter 2000).

Using qualitative evidence in health promotion: application of the nominal group technique

Responding to changes in health policy in Australia that require consumer involvement in planning health promotion programmes (to ensure both relevance and appropriateness), Twible (1992) reported on research that explored the concerns, attitudes, beliefs and values of consumers in planning a health promotion project for war veterans and their widows. In so doing, Twible (1992) used the nominal group technique.

Twible's project team surveyed more than 400 people over a 6-week period, using groups of about 20 people on average and enabling everyone who had expressed an interest in the research to become involved.

Unlike much research, which neglects to distribute findings to those subjected to the research, Twible's group was able to provide study results to the participants before the groups dispersed, thereby reinforcing the importance and value of what had been accomplished. Convening groups in diverse geographical areas enabled specific local concerns to be identified. Twible (1992) noted that use of this qualitative method of research generated issues not previously raised in the literature, demonstrating that compilation of a literature-informed questionnaire would have failed to address some issues of importance to the consumer group in question.

Although rarely reported in the rehabilitation literature, Twible's (1992) study suggests the value of the nominal group technique in identifying client-generated issues, thereby contributing to a credible and relevant evidence base with which to inform subsequent practice.

USING QUALITATIVE EVIDENCE AS A BASIS FOR EVIDENCE-BASED PRACTICE: THE SYSTEMATIC REVIEW

Central to traditional concepts of evidence-based practice, the systematic review is a rigorous and explicit research method that aims to locate, appraise and synthesize the available research evidence pertaining to a specific research question and to evaluate the quality of the studies using predetermined criteria (Bannigan 1997, Brown & Burns 2001). Systematic reviews thus yield conclusions with which to guide practice by assembling and critically examining the results from many studies. Brown & Burns (2001), for example, demonstrated the effectiveness of this method by documenting a systematic review of quantitative research into the efficacy of neurodevelopmental treatment in paediatrics. In the nursing literature, Beck (2002) describes a meta-synthesis of qualitative research that amalgamated the findings of several studies to reveal shared findings, thus providing a richer understanding of an issue than is possible from the results of one study. Other researchers have performed systematic reviews that employ a quantitative meta-analysis in concert with a qualitative meta-synthesis (e.g. Higginson et al 2002). Recent recognition of the role of qualitative evidence to systematic reviews by the British National Health Service Centre for Reviews and Dissemination prompted Dixon-Woods & Fitzpatrick (2001, p. 765) to observe: 'The argument for giving a place to qualitative research in systematic reviews seems to have been won'.

The Cochrane Collaboration, an international network of researchers who compile, critically appraise and disseminate systematic reviews of the effects of healthcare interventions, contributes to the Cochrane Library, which publishes systematic reviews in an electronic database to enable clinicians to utilize the best available knowledge in clinical practice. Originally concerned solely with research evidence derived from studies using a quantitative methodology, the Cochrane Collaboration now recognizes qualitative evidence as a legitimate source of knowledge, particularly in determining the *appropriateness* of interventions to individual patients.

The Cochrane Qualitative Methods Group maintains a website (see Further reading), which includes a bibliographical database of references. The website describes the current areas of activity of the Methods Group, such as: 'demonstrating the value of including evidence from qualitative research and process evaluations into systematic reviews' and 'developing and disseminating methodological standards' (accessed 28.11.02).

Systematic reviews, by definition, require defined standards for evaluating the quality of research, prompting Popay et al (1998) to call for a hierarchy of qualitative research evidence (see also Dixon-Woods & Fitzpatrick 2001). Such a hierarchy would be determined by certain standards of rigour, and it is to the assessment of rigour in qualitative research that we now turn.

CRITICALLY EVALUATING QUALITATIVE RESEARCH

If qualitative research is to provide rigorous and convincing evidence on which to base practice, it must be capable of withstanding critical scrutiny regarding the quality and relevance of researchers' work (Kuzel & Engel 2001). Agencies that fund health-related research require guidance on how to evaluate qualitative research (Devers 1999), and practitioners need sufficient information from which to evaluate the strength and plausibility of the evidence reported, and its relevance to their practice situations (Hammell 2002).

The procedure for critiquing qualitative research is not one of judging rigid adherence to rules or specific prescriptive criteria (Hasselkus 1995), but is a process of weighing the various elements of the research in an effort to determine their appropriateness given the purpose and context of the study. Although qualitative research entails an inherently creative process, this cannot preclude rigour of both research process and reporting. Rehabilitation research is undertaken for the benefit of clients and with the goal of informing theory and improving practice, and it is therefore incumbent upon the profession to evaluate all inquiry with attention to how dependably it might achieve these goals (Hammell 2002, Kuzel & Engel 2001). 'This is especially important for research undertaken into issues of health and social care, where research can – and should – have consequences for those people we study' (Hammell 2002, p. 182).

Criteria for evaluating the quality of qualitative research have been explored elsewhere (e.g. Carpenter & Hammell 2000, Hammell 2002). Box 11.1 gives a summary and should be tailored to suit the nature and purpose of each specific study.

It is important to reiterate that the information in Box 11.1 constitutes a summary, at best, and that these criteria may be satisfied in different ways, congruent with the nature and purpose of each study. The goal must be to achieve a high standard of qualitative research that will have meaning and relevance to the groups we study, contribute to the knowledge base of our professions, and justify the

---

Box 11.1 Framework of guidelines for evaluating qualitative research (see Carpenter & Hammell 2000, Hammell 2002, Popay et al 1998)

- *Relevance, usefulness and appropriateness of the study, methodology and methods* – What and who prompted the study and why? Are the study and methods supported by a thorough and comprehensive literature review?
- *Privileging of lay accounts* – Are the participants' perspectives and meanings presented and privileged? How was respondent validation encouraged? What were the ethical implications of the study? Are the participants comfortable with how their experiences will be used? Where will findings be presented? Whose point of view is used to represent the findings? Does the research narrow the gap between 'lay' and 'expert' knowledge, thus providing the basis for evidence-based client choice? (Brechin & Sidell 2000).
- *Evidence of typicality and transferability* – Although the purpose of qualitative research is primarily to describe a particular experience or context, not to generalize this to others (Sandelowski 1986), if qualitative findings are to guide and facilitate the evaluation of practice in a diversity of settings researchers need to provide information concerning the *transferability* of the findings. This pertains to the degree to which the application of findings to other contexts and settings, or with other groups, can be judged. Transferability is dependent upon information concerning the representativeness of the informants and details

of the research context and setting (Lincoln & Guba 1985).
- *Evidence of theoretical or purposeful sampling* – Was sampling appropriate and relevant, given the nature and purpose of the study? How were participants recruited? What were their characteristics?
- *Evidence of data quality* – What were the data collection methods, process and mode of documentation? Were the methods appropriate to the research purpose? Were multiple methods used and were these choices justified? How were discrepancies arising from different methods addressed? Was the process flexible? How was the length of time spent in data collection determined?
- *Evidence of theoretical and conceptual rigour* – How were the findings identified from the data? How was analysis undertaken? Does a decision trail justify the interpretations? How do the findings relate to, contest or further existing theories?
- *Evidence of critique of power* – Is the researcher's role, social and philosophical positioning critically analysed? To what extent were the study participants enabled to participate in the research process, from design through analysis and evaluation of findings?
- *Evidence to support conclusions* – What did the study conclude and are the conclusions justified in relation to the data collected and consistent with the findings? What are the implications of the findings and how might the findings be used?

---

role of qualitative research in informing the client-centred, evidence-based practice of our professions (Hammell 2002).

MIXING METHODS: POTENTIALS AND POSSIBILITIES

Most researchers acknowledge the futility of dogmatic allegiance to either qualitative or quantitative methods, recognizing that a research 'question' or issue should determine the methods used for investigation (Morgan 1998). In many instances, the question and context require the use of both qualitative *and* quantitative methods, and, while it may be unrealistic to expect expertise in both methods, rehabilitation clinicians and researchers need to be well versed in both paradigms in order to be able to critique the research literature and to design and implement studies utilizing mixed methods that will address clinical questions and more adequately inform practice.

Although mixing methods traditionally meant treating qualitative methods as somehow subservient to the quantitative paradigm, more recent acknowledgement of the variety with which these methods can be combined, coupled with a greater degree of sophistication and knowledge among researchers about the strengths of the different paradigms, has enabled the two methods to be appropriately combined to address complex research issues. As Miller & Crabtree (2000, p. 610) emphasize, use of qualitative methods in concert with qualitative ones enables the recovery of 'the missing evidence … the richness and depth of what "effectiveness" means' and exploration of 'the human implications of rationing and cost issues'. They assert the need for participatory, collaborative, multi-method approaches to clinical research to ensure that research findings are not alienated from their clinical context.

It is important to recognize that simply adding a few interviews to a quantitative study constitutes neither qualitative research nor mixed-method research. Qualitative research reflects particular epistemological assumptions, and demands the same respect for methodological rigour as does quantitative research (see previous section). Increasingly, qualitative and quantitative methods are being used in elegant combination to comprehend and address the complex issues of health care more thoroughly. This final section will briefly outline some of the ways in which methods can be mixed to address particular research issues.

Sequential design

Probably the most common form of mixed methods, the sequential design calls for one method to inform the other. Typically, qualitative research precedes quantitative research by exploring both the context and the meanings of an issue to the study participants, and thereafter identifying hypotheses and variables that might be measured and statistically analysed, using language that will be clear to study respondents (Black 1994, Miller & Crabtree 2000, Morgan 1998). Indeed, Pope & Mays (1995) claim that qualitative research is a *prerequisite* of good quantitative research, 'particularly in areas that have received little previous investigation' (p. 42). Michael Curtin & Emily Jaramazovic (Ch. 10) used the insights gained from focus groups to inform the development of a questionnaire. This mixed-method design ensured that the questionnaire would enable exploration of those issues clinicians considered to be important, thus ensuring relevance. Conversely, Mallinson (2002) employed qualitative methods to evaluate patients' experiences with an existing quantitative research tool – the Short-Form 36 Health Status Questionnaire. Mallinson's findings prompted her to observe: 'without more assessment of people's understandings of survey questions it is difficult to see how one can establish their validity as subjective health measures' (p. 20). Thus, qualitative research can enhance both the accuracy and relevance of quantitative research (Black 1994).

Frequently, a quantitative survey may be used to discover the scale of a problem (such as the incidence of domestic abuse experienced by disabled women) and a qualitative study may follow, to explore the factors contributing to disabled women's social isolation and perceived difficulties with accessing support or refuge. Or, a qualitative study may be undertaken to provide explanations for unexpected or unexplained findings from a quantitative study (Black 1994).

Concurrent design

Concurrent designs may be used to explore both what happens (quantitative methods) and why, and in which specific contexts (qualitative methods). This use of different research methods can provide a form of triangulation: testing and validating the findings from one method with the findings of another (Pope & Mays 1995). Clinical trials are enhanced when researchers simultaneously conduct qualitative studies that help them both to understand the clinical trial process and to explain why an intervention does or does not work (Miller & Crabtree 2000). Although researchers frequently choose to ignore findings that appear contradictory (thus imposing their own judgement on the plausibility and importance of the various findings), triangulation requires thorough analysis and interpretation of discrepancies to enhance understanding of data that do not immediately appear consistent (McLaughlin 1991).

Morgan (1998) observed that health researchers have a particular interest in the possibilities of combining quantitative and qualitative methods because human health is such a complex issue and because the different research approaches are able to tease out and illuminate different dimensions of this complexity. For rehabilitation researchers, who recognize that occupations and functional movements are necessarily context specific and imbued with subjective meanings, the choice to enhance quantitative studies by incorporating qualitative evidence will have a special imperative.

CONCLUDING THOUGHTS

Occupational and physical therapists recognize the growing social, political and ethical imperatives to justify their approaches to intervention and service delivery with reference to an evidence base. Therapists are also required to ensure that their interventions are informed by a sound theoretical base, that is, by theory supported by research evidence. The examples in this book have illustrated some of the many ways in which qualitative research can contribute to the generation of relevant and useful research to inform theory, practice, research and service delivery. Philosophically compatible with a client-centred ethic, qualitative methods enable researchers to identify ways in which therapy interventions and modes of service delivery may be better crafted to meet the needs and priorities of clients.

This book has advocated a client-centred approach to knowledge development, argued for the need to employ qualitative methods to address the issues of importance to clients and clinicians, and has supported these contentions with evidence derived from nine research studies.

REFERENCES

Abberley P 1995 Disabling ideology in Health and Welfare: the case of occupational therapy. Disability and Society 10(2):221–232

Alcoff L 1991 The problem of speaking for others. Cultural Critique Winter:5–31

Bannigan K 1997 Clinical effectiveness: systematic reviews and evidence-based practice in occupational therapy. British Journal of Occupational Therapy 60(11):479–483

Barclay-Goddard R, Strock A 2001 A collaborative approach to learning needs assessment using the Delphi technique. Physiotherapy Canada Summer:190–194

Beck C 2002 Mothering multiples: a meta-synthesis of qualitative research. American Journal of Maternal Child Nursing 27(4):214–221

Black N 1994 Why we need qualitative research. Journal of Epidemiology and Community Health 48:425–426

Bodenhamer E, Achterberg-Lawlis J, Kevorkian G, Belanus A, Cofer J 1983 Staff and patient perceptions of the psychosocial concerns of spinal cord injured persons. American Journal of Physical Medicine 62(4):182–193

Bodiam C 1999 The use of the Canadian Occupational Performance Measure for the assessment of outcome on a neurorehabilitation unit. British Journal of Occupational Therapy 62(3):123–126

Brechin A, Sidell M 2000 Ways of knowing. In: Gomm R, Davies C (eds) Using evidence in health and social care. Sage and the Open University, London; pp. 3–25

Brown GT, Burns SA 2001 The efficacy of neurodevelopmental treatment in paediatrics: a systematic review. British Journal of Occupational Therapy 64(5):235–244

Canadian Association of Occupational Therapists, Health Services Directorate 1983 Guidelines for the client-centred practice of occupational therapy. Health Services Directorate, Ottawa

Carpenter C, Hammell KW 2000 Evaluating qualitative research. In: Hammell KW, Carpenter C, Dyck I (eds) Using qualitative research. A practical introduction for occupational and physical therapists. Churchill Livingstone, Edinburgh; pp. 107–119

Clark C, Scott E, Krupa T 1993 Involving clients in programme evaluation and research: a new methodology. Canadian Journal of Occupational Therapy 60(4):192–199

Corring DJ 1999 The missing perspective on client-centred care. OT Now Jan–Feb:8–10

Cott CA, Finch E, Gasner D, Yoshida K, Thomas S, Verrier M 1995 The movement continuum theory of physical therapy. Physiotherapy Canada 47(2):87–95

Dale AE 1995 A research study exploring the patient's view of quality of life using the case study method. Journal of Advanced Nursing 22:1128–1134

Davidson I, Waters K 2000 Physiotherapists working with stoke patients: a national survey. Physiotherapy 86(2):69–80

Davidson L, Stayner D, Lambert S, Smith P, Sledge W 1997 Phenomenological and participatory research on schizophrenia: recovering the person in theory and practice. Journal of Social Issues 53(4):767–784

Devers KJ 1999 How will we know 'good' qualitative research when we see it? Beginning the dialogue in health services research. Health Services Research 34:1153–1188

Dixon-Woods M, Fitzpatrick R 2001 Qualitative research in systematic reviews. British Medical Journal 323:765–766

Eisenberg M, Saltz C 1991 Quality of life among aging spinal cord injured persons: long term rehabilitation outcomes. Paraplegia 29:514–520

Ernst FA 1987 Contrasting perceptions of distress by research personnel and their spinal cord injured subjects. American Journal of Physical Medicine 66(1):12–15

Fischer D, Stewart A, Bloch D, Lorig K, Laurent D, Holman H 1999 Capturing the patient's view of change as a clinical outcome measure. Journal of the American Medical Association 282(12):1157–1162

Gill TM, Feinstein AR 1994 A critical appraisal of the quality of quality-of-life measurements. Journal of the American Medical Association 272(8):619–626

Hammell KW 2001 Using qualitative research to inform the client-centred evidence-based practice of occupational therapy. British Journal of Occupational Therapy 64(5):228–234

Hammell KW 2002 Informing client-centred practice through qualitative inquiry: evaluating the quality of qualitative research. British Journal of Occupational Therapy 65(4):175–184

Hammell KW 2003 The rehabilitation process. In: Stokes M, Ashburn A (eds) Physical management in neurological rehabilitation. 2nd edn. Harcourt, Edinburgh (in press)

Hammell KW, Carpenter C 2000 Introduction to qualitative research in occupational and physical therapy. In: Hammell KW, Carpenter C, Dyck I (eds) Using qualitative research: a practical introduction for occupational and physical therapists. Churchill Livingstone, Edinburgh; pp. 1–12

Hasselkus BR 1995 Beyond ethnography: expanding our understanding and criteria for qualitative research. Occupational Therapy Journal of Research 15(2):75–84

Higginson IJ, Finlay I, Goodwin D et al 2002 Do hospital-based palliative teams improve care for patients or families at the end of life? Journal of Pain and Symptom Management 23(2):96–106

Ilott I, White E 2001 2001 College of Occupational Therapists' Research and Development Strategic Vision and Action Plan. British Journal of Occupational Therapy 64(6):270–277

Jones J, Hunter D 2000 Using the Delphi and nominal group technique in health services research. In: Pope C, Mays N (eds) Qualitative research in healthcare. 2nd edn. BMJ Books, London; pp. 40–49

Jorgensen P 2000 Concepts of body and health in physiotherapy: the meaning of the social/cultural aspects of life. Physiotherapy Theory and Practice 16:105–115

Kuzel AJ, Engel JD 2001 Some pragmatic thoughts about evaluating qualitative health research. In: Morse J, Swanson J, Kuzel A (eds) The nature of qualitative evidence. Sage, London; pp. 114–138

Laliberte-Rudman D, Yu B, Scott E, Pajouhandeh P 2000 Exploration of the perspectives of persons with schizophrenia regarding quality of life. American Journal of Occupational Therapy 54:137–147

Law M 1998a Does client-centred practice make a difference? In: Law M (ed) Client-centered occupational therapy. Slack, Thorofare, NJ; pp. 19–27

Law M 1998b Preface. In: Law M (ed) Client-centered occupational therapy. Slack, Thorofare, NJ: pp. xv–xvi

Law M, Baptiste S, Carswell A, McColl MA, Polatajko H, Pollock N 1998 The Canadian Occupational Performance Measure. 3rd edn. CAOT Publications, Ottawa

Lincoln YS, Guba EG 1985 Naturalistic inquiry. Sage, Beverley Hills, CA

MacDonald C, Houghton P, Cox P, Bartlett D 2001 Consensus on physical therapy professional behaviours. Physiotherapy Canada Summer:212–218, 222

Mallinson S 2002 Listening to respondents: a qualitative assessment of the Short-Form 36 Health Status Questionnaire. Social Science and Medicine 54:11–21

McLaughlin E 1991 Oppositional poverty: the quantitative/qualitative divide and other dichotomies. Sociological Review 39:292–308

Miles-Tapping C, Dyck A, Brunham S, Simpson E, Barber L 1990 Canadian therapists' priorities for clinical research. Physical Therapy 70(7):448–454

Miller WL, Crabtree BF 2000 Clinical research. In: Denzin N, Lincoln Y (eds) Handbook of qualitative research. 2nd edn. Sage, London; pp. 607–631

Morgan DL 1998 Practical strategies for combining qualitative and quantitative methods: applications to health research. Qualitative Health Research 8(3):362–376

Needham G, Oliver S 1998 Involving service users. In: Bury T, Mead J (eds) Evidence-based healthcare. A practical guide for therapists. Butterworth-Heinemann, Oxford; pp. 85–103

Oliver M 1996 Understanding disability: from theory to practice. Macmillan, Basingstoke

Popay J, Rogers A, Williams G 1998 Rationale and standards for the systematic review of qualitative literature in health services research. Qualitative Health Research 8(3):341–351

Pope C, Mays N 1995 Reaching the parts other methods cannot reach: an introduction to qualitative methods in health and health services research. British Medical Journal 311:42–45

Pope C, Mays N 2000 Qualitative research in health care. 2nd edn. BMJ Books, London

Ray LD, Mayan M 2001 Who decides what counts as evidence? In: Morse J, Swanson J, Kuzel A (eds) The nature

of qualitative evidence. Sage, Thousand Oaks, CA; pp. 50–73

Richardson B 1999 Professional development. 2. Professional knowledge and situated learning in the workplace. Physiotherapy 85(9):467–474

Sackett D, Strauss S, Richardson W, Rosenberg W, Hayes R 2000 Evidence-based medicine. How to practice and teach EBM. 2nd edn. Churchill Livingstone, Edinburgh

Sandelowski M 1986 The problem of rigor in qualitative research. Advances in Nursing Science 8(3):27–37

Smith DE 1990 Texts, facts and femininity: exploring the relations of ruling. Routledge, London

Stephenson S, Wiles R 2000 Advantages and disadvantages of the home setting for therapy: views of patients and therapists. British Journal of Occupational Therapy 63(2):59–64

Stratford P, Gill C, Westaway M, Binkley J 1995 Assessing disability and change on individual patients: a report of a patient-specific measure. Physiotherapy Canada 47(4):258–262

Sumsion T 1998 The Delphi technique: an adaptive research tool. British Journal of Occupational Therapy 61(4):153–156

Sumsion T 1999 A study to determine a British occupational therapy definition of client-centred practice. British Journal of Occupational Therapy 62(2):52–58

Thomas C, Parry A 1996 Research on users' views about stroke services: towards an empowerment research paradigm or more of the same? Physiotherapy 82(1):6–12

Townsend E 1996 Institutional ethnography: a method for showing how the context shapes practice. Occupational Therapy Journal of Research 16(3):179–199

Twible RL 1992 Consumer participation in planing health promotion programmes: a case study using the nominal group technique. Australian Occupational Therapy Journal 39(2):13–18

Walker AM 1994 A Delphi study of research priorities in the clinical practice of physiotherapy. Physiotherapy 80(4):205–207

Walker MF, Drummond A, Gatt J, Sackley C 2000 Occupational therapy for stroke patients: a survey of current practice. British Journal of Occupational Therapy 63(8):367–372

Westaway MD, Stratford PW, Binkley JM 1998 The Patient-Specific Functional Scale: validation of its use in persons with neck dysfunction. Journal of Orthopaedic and Sports Physical Therapy 27(5):331–338

Whiteford GE, Wilcock AA 2000 Cultural relativism: occupation and independence reconsidered. Canadian Journal of Occupational Therapy 67(5):324–336

Woolsey R 1985 Rehabilitation outcome following spinal cord injury. Archives of Neurology 42:116–119

FURTHER READING

Cochrane Qualitative Methods Group. Online. Available: http://mysite.freeserve.com/Cochrane_Qual_Method/index.htm

Law M (ed) 2002 Evidence-based rehabilitation: a guide to practice. Slack, Thorofare, NJ

Morse JM, Swanson JM, Kuzel AJ 2001 The nature of qualitative evidence. Sage, London

Index

Page numbers in **bold** indicate figures and tables